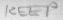

EAST END DOC
Hospices and the dying

Richard Lamerton

Illustrations by
Brian Tutt

LUTTERWORTH PRESS
Cambridge

362.1

British Library Cataloguing in Publication Data
Lamerton, Richard
  East end doc.
  1. Hospices (Terminal care)
  I. Title
362.1'75   R726.8

ISBN 0-7188-2624-8

First published 1986

Lutterworth Press
7 All Saints' Passage
Cambridge CB2 3LS

Typeset in Monophoto Bembo by
Vision Typesetting, Manchester

Made and printed in Great Britain by the Guernsey Press Co. Ltd.,
Guernsey, Channel Islands.

TO
Harriet, Clare and Antonia

CONTENTS

Acknowledgements   vi

1   What's all this about, then?   1

2   Early days   10

3   Sister Bridget   12

4   The team grows   21

5   Care of dying Cockneys   24

6   Hospice care is family care   33

7   Professional hazards   46

8   Letting people be themselves   49

9   Discovering how to use the drugs   52

10   Much more than drugs   58

11   'Telling'   67

12   Euthanasia   75

13   Immigrant patients   82

14   Volunteers – community support   90

15   A international model – the Hospice Movement   95

A selection of British hospices   99

Books I would recommend   105

ACKNOWLEDGEMENTS

I worked for thirteen years as a doctor in Cockney Country, east of Tower Bridge, trying to find out the basic principles of good care for people who were dying of cancer. In doing the work, and later in writing this book about it because my friends told me I just must write about it, I was helped by a host of wonderful people. The nuns of St Joseph's Hospice, Dame Cicely Saunders, my teacher and mentor, and the great team of nurses, doctors and social workers in the Macmillan Service were all woven into the tapestry. Many have helped me, and it would be almost churlish to pick one out, but Harriet Copperman must have special mention as a particular source of inspiration, encouragement and practical help.

The ones who taught me all I have to offer and who entranced me for thirteen glorious years of alternate laughter and eye-pricking tears were our patients. Of course I have changed all the names of the families whose bereavements I have peeped into, and where anyone would be still recognisable, I have changed other details as well. But the book is just an account of my experiences as a physician in East London.

1

WHAT'S ALL THIS ABOUT, THEN?

People ask, 'Don't you find it dreadfully depressing, looking after dying people all the time?' I tell them about Mr Cardew.

'I can't bear to see 'im suffer like this. 'E'll 'ave to go into 'ospital,' Mrs Cardew had said to me when I first saw him. She was a dumpy little old lady with straggly hair and a tubular blue smock. Spindly ankle-stalks disappeared into fluffy pink slippers with a hole in the toe. She was pulling off a dirty apron and turned a woeful face to me. No teeth. Faded grey eyes sunk in red sockets. Wrinkles like a tree bark. How did a lovely young woman ever get so battered and shrunken? 'I can't take any more doc.' Tears filled her eyes and she peered into a misty distance across the estate towards Spitalfields Church. 'We was married in there. Such a fine figure of a man 'e was. I don't know why this should 'appen I'm sure I dont – 'e was always a clean living man . . . I can't watch it anymore.'

Watch what? The family doctor, a kindly Indian run off his feet with a list of patients twice the national average, had referred Mr Cardew to us because his case perplexed him. His cancer pain was out of control and it was becoming impossible to treat it because he was vomiting. He had eaten nothing for three weeks. Now he was confused and had started messing the bed. His wife's arthritis was playing up, she had no bed linen left and was weeping and depressed because in his confusion he was becoming abusive to her.

She shuffled dejectedly before me and stood helplessly at the door of the stale-smelling bedroom. There lay Mr Cardew, half uncovered, unshaven, wheezing weakly, with diarrhoea down his legs and under his finger nails. Any movement, even coughing, made him give a hoarse shout as showers of pain

1

from the cancer in his spine flooded down his buttocks and legs.

But through trained eyes the problem quickly resolved itself into a series of diagnoses, all of which I made from the bed end. In my notes I wrote a list of his urgent needs – morphine, a bath, an enema, some clean bedding. We could provide them all the same day.

'I'll tell you what, love. Give it two more days and see if you still can't cope. And if you can't, he can go to St Joseph's.' She stared at me disbelievingly. 'I'll stop his pain by tonight, and the vomiting. There will be a nurse in later today, and every day as long as you need her. And you won't have any more messed beds – that's only due to his constipation which nurse will deal with today.' We had to visit twice more that day because the nurse couldn't deal with the drastic constipation. So I had to come back to give him an anaesthetic.

After my two-day deadline Mr Cardew welcomed me from his armchair in front of 'Match of the Day'. Mrs Cardew's deep sorrowful eyes were full of wonder and gratitude because he was back in his right mind and, best of all possible blessings, he had eaten the lunch she prepared. His pain was gone and his cough was subsiding as a result of the medications. He did not remember much from the last week, but he did seem to recognise me. 'It's nice of you to call in, Father,' he said. I wondered what sort of a priest he thought it was that stuck a finger in his backside and provided commodes!

Mr Cardew lived another two weeks. His wife coped with most of his needs and felt very secure because we came every day and a neighbour offered her phone, day or night, in case we were needed. He died peacefully and easily in his own bed with her asleep beside him, sad but prepared. At Christmas she scraped together and sent us a fiver.

Now how could you be depressed doing work like that? One glorious success story after another. You see, for a hospice team a good death is a success. To start with frightened, isolated people in pain, and transform the situation to one of relief and self-reliance is enormously satisfying. This work is never depressing if the attitude to it is right. On the contrary, it is delightful. Because of the way someone's priorities may fall into place as death approaches, a new calm comes to them, a greater consideration for those around them, and often a gentle confidence. We are daily seeing mankind at its best. Our faith in people is constantly renewed. And, unexpectedly perhaps, as I hope this book makes evident, caring for people like this can be *fun*.

It isn't death that alarms people so much as dying. Here is a letter I received from her daughter after one of our patients died. I haven't included it here to throw flowers at the staff, but because I think it expresses exactly what we were trying to do:

Dear Dr Lamerton,

I wish to thank you and your nurses for the care and attention you gave to my mother through her recent illness.

I was desperate for help and you didn't stint it, you and your nurses gave me the courage to carry on with a job I would never have dreamed I was capable of. I cannot speak highly enough of your organisation, and more power to your elbow.

Anyway, once again

Thank you all for your help and God bless you all.

Yours sincerely

As a medical student I was horrified at our professional incompetence with dying patients. There has been a little improvement in the twenty years since then, but only a little. So a few of us – doctors, nurses and social workers – decided to specialise in the needs of families caring for someone who is dying, and in trying to serve those needs.

A few orders of nuns – notably the Irish Sisters of Charity – began the work in former generations, but it was Dame Cicely Saunders at St Christopher's Hospice in South London who really formulated the principles of good modern terminal care. She pointed out how inadequate was our pain control, how physical distress was not treated as important, how patronising were doctors who would not let patients discuss their fears and how bereavement was not seen as a doctor's concern. All that is slowly changing, thank heaven.

Don't get me wrong, mind you: most people, even if they have cancer, have a peaceful death with no distressing complications. And most could die at home. Even in socially-deprived East London we had more than two-thirds of our patients dying at home. All we did was to support the family so that they could cope, as the letter on page 3 shows. If they could not cope, there was always a bed in the St Joseph's Hospice. At all costs we wanted to avoid a hospital death. (In fact, the *cost* of hospice care is always less than that in a hospital.)

Even a good hospital, with committed, caring staff, is not the best place to die. It is often too noisy and busy. There is a constant turnover of nursing and junior medical staff, many of whom have not had the opportunity to examine their own negative attitudes to dying patients. Hospitals usually are not family-orientated, nor equipped for the subsequent bereavement: they simply don't have the necessary experience or skills.

One study of thirteen patients in pain in a famous London teaching hospital showed that only four of them received anything like relief.[1] Doctors and nurses gave hopelessly inaccurate descriptions of the site, nature and duration of the pain. Severe and continuous pain was found in one-fifth of patients who died in South London hospitals.[2] Furthermore, it was shown in Canada that pain-killers used in a hospice unit were more effective than the same drugs used in a general hospital ward, because the environment was more supportive.[3] In 1982 more than a quarter of the families of someone

4

who had died in hospital in Sheffield complained of having found an uncaring attitude among the staff.[4]

Family doctors often do no better. In 1980 a third of our patients were referred to us with severe untreated constipation and 5 per cent with a total bowel blockage from constipation. Two-thirds had pain, and one in ten of those needed only mild pain killers administered regularly to relieve them completely. The South London study showed that in the week before death, more than a quarter of the patients who stayed at home had severe and continuous pain.

In Sheffield in 1982 twice as many dying people had uncontrolled pain and bowel problems as the GP was aware of, and there were about four times as many with insomnia and bedsores.

A quarter of the families regretted insufficient district nursing visits. In 1982 there were still 57 per cent of Sheffield GPs who would not visit the bereaved. Nevertheless Sheffield is probably better than most because of the ten years of energetic teaching which Professor Wilkes devoted to the topic of caring for the dying.

A survey in Manchester in 1982 found that only 10 per cent of dying patients received regular follow-up from their GPs. In Edinburgh in 1980 a quarter of patients who were incontinent were receiving no home nursing visits, and of dying patients who lived alone, less than half had been visited by a district nurse before the hospice team was called in. In 1983 the Consumers' Association, in a nationwide survey, found that over a quarter of out-of-hours attempts to contact a doctor resulted in failure. All these figures help to make the point that there's room for improvement. Much of this distress can be relieved by a trained and enthusiastic team – hence the need for hospices.

The hospice movement wasn't some boffin's bright idea. It was a practical response to obvious needs. No better answer has yet been devised; it leaves the patient and his family free to behave as they would like, while offering any help they might need, either at home or in a special in-patient environment.

You can't beat common sense and a willingness to serve.

It was an enterprising nurse called Barbara McNulty who first began to visit people at home from St Christopher's Hospice in South London. We in East London followed suit in 1971, eventually building up a team of specialist district nurses. Before long we were in it up to our neck. Annual reports recorded the variety of activities:

1976 We removed stitches from the head of one gentleman who fell off a bus, inserted many catheters and gave many hundreds of enemas. Along with patients being admitted we took in a dog, a cat and two canaries, and rehoused a family of kittens. We found a job for one patient's son [he's now a qualified lab technician] and attended another son's wedding [who now has three kids!]. Four visits to patients by spouses in prison were organised. One old husband and wife from Islington were both admitted to the Hospice simultaneously so that they could stay together. They died within a month of one another. We helped a lady to write her will. When a night nurse was not available, one of the Sisters sat all night with a patient.

1977 In co-operation with Michael Sobell House, the Oxford Hospice, we made a film to teach doctors about pain control. Medical students and visitors from all over the globe came to see us at work . . . from the USA, Norway, Japan, Australia, New Zealand, Holland, Eire and Germany. Dr Lamerton made another lecture tour of the USA and has seen American and Japanese editions of his textbook *Care of the Dying* published.[5]

We lent our canary to cheer up two patients, as well as a television [which blew up], cassettes of music and short stories, and a couple of wigs. Our new portable suction apparatus has proved very valuable for some patients. Team members witnessed two patients' wills. Three married couples were both admitted to our care. We took two patients to Lourdes.

1978   Two patients came to the clinic regularly in order to be able to practise on the Hospice chapel organ.

We gave one blood transfusion and emptied a hydrocele. Two of our patients were under seven years of age.

1979   Four patients had landlord troubles, which we helped them to fight, two were blind, three had shingles. Every Thursday afternoon the clinic provided some social life for groups of patients who would otherwise be housebound. One hundred and nine patients made 425 attendances at the clinic this year . . . which depends upon our volunteer drivers to bring patients in from all over the area. Volunteers kept the tea flowing and made the whole event a social occasion . . . .

We syringed ears, gave rectal infusions, dressed ulcers, manipulated spines, gave bladder washouts, and lent people electric fires, food liquidizers, armchairs and a television [which was later stolen].

1980   We found ourselves being filmed by the BBC for 'Brass Tacks' and by Granada for 'World in Action'.

'Half the team trundled to Wales to the wedding of Dr James, our previous Registrar . . . and for our works outing this year we took our volunteers to the Westminster Cathedral Carol Service.

For the rapid retrieval of statistical information we transferred records onto a punched-card system.

The other main area of work is the follow-up of families, relatives or friends of the patient. There is often a great deal to be sorted out practically, for example the patient may have died intestate, or a wife might not know how to put money in the meter because her husband always did it, or a husband finds that ironing a shirt defeats him. It is surprising to discover how many women are frightened to get on a bus on their own. The MOT testing of cars or hanging of curtains is strange territory. Equally the rigours of a supermarket queue and the mysteries of the deep-freeze are problems for men left to fend for themselves.

Alongside these practical considerations, surviving relat-

7

ives often feel a sense of deep loss and despair. A sizeable proportion of these contemplate suicide, many more talk of feeling unable to carry on. It is our job to care for them during this time until the overwhelming sense of grief makes way for an absorbed sadness, that no longer dictates a life pattern, but becomes part of it . . . . Most of this work is undertaken by visiting at home, but we also have a club which meets fortnightly where bereaved people can meet and talk and make new friends, who understand how they feel.

1981   Monty Modlin launched a fund-raising drive for us in Newham pubs, bless him, with an unforgettably atrocious yarn about an ablutions attendant on Park Lane.

Each week we have a joint meeting with members of the Hackney Hospital Oncology Unit team, and with the London Hospital Radiotherapy Department.

Our Jobst compression pump for swollen limbs was much used. Ears were syringed, IV anti-cancer drugs were given . . . a dislocated shoulder was reduced and sutures were removed.

1982   The physiotherapist: 'I have been called upon to treat chest infections and painful joints, to mobilise the bedridden, to make or arrange for the making of splints and the provision of aids and adaptations, and to teach families how they can most easily lift and handle their sick relatives.'

A Bangladeshi gentleman pulled at our heart strings and had us agree to enable him, so we thought, to leave hospital and die in his adopted home in East London. However, after a few days in his own bed and with some changes in his medication he showed more signs of living than dying. Some time later his final ambition was reached when he set off for his native Bangladesh.

But I'm jumping the gun. First I must tell you how all this was started.

Notes

1. J.M. Hunt *et al.*, 'Patients with protracted pain', *The Journal of Medical Ethics*, **III**, 2 (1977), p. 61.

2. C.M. Parkes, 'Home or hospital?', *The Journal of the Royal College of General Practitioners*, **XXVIII**, 186 (1978), p. 19.

3. R. Melzack *et al.*, 'The Brompton mixture', *Canadian Medical Association Journal*, **CXV**, July 17 (1976), p. 125.

4. E. Wilkes, Scargill Hospices Conference, 7 June 1983.

5. Reprinted by Penguin Books in 1980.

2

EARLY DAYS

I had been very troubled by the first dying patient I met as a medical student. People wanted to reassure me that I would get used to it and be able to cope with death. But it wasn't death that bothered me. It never has. Death's no problem – it's the manner of dying. The man was so haunted. So isolated. He complained of pain every time I saw him, but when I fussed I was made to feel small – he already had heroin for the pain, did I want to turn him into an addict?

Then a doctor died in the surgical ward. They even printed a false laboratory report to convince him his operation had been more successful than it had. He was lonely and angry. He was no fool, and could see perfectly well what was happening, but couldn't talk to anyone.

This all bewildered me. No one answered the patients' questions, and the subject of death was avoided or ignored. What a relief then, to go to a lecture by Dr Cicely Saunders. I was disillusioned, finding that medical school was not fulfilling any of my hopes. So much of what we were witnessing seemed to miss the point. Research, careers, status were the gods. Service was out of fashion. Then this doctor from a 'hospice' gave a lecture called 'Care of the Dying'. She seemed to be from another planet. I had long ceased to be dazzled by medical technology. We had our successes, but they were so obviously limited. Yet here was somone who, like me, was concerned for all those we had NOT cured. She urged us to communicate with our patients, to face up to subjects like death and to care for the 'visitors' as well as the patients in the hospital. It all sounds obvious now – it is all fashionable now – but in 1962 it was like the clarion call of revolution.

'It's all very well for you, Dr Saunders,' one pompous consultant had said to her. 'But you're a doctor with time, lots of time. We're busy hospital doctors, and we couldn't possibly spend so much time on all this listening you're talking about.' In fact, at that point in her life Dr Saunders was coping with something like double the work load of the consultant questioning her. So I was interested to see what she would say. Her reply, so simple, so humbly offered, redirected my whole life. 'Oh no, doctor. Time isn't a question of length. It's a question of depth, isn't it? It's how completely you listen that counts.'

From that day on I wanted to work with Dr Saunders. As soon as my training was complete I asked her if she needed a junior doctor. Her reply was 'You're just what we've been praying for.' She had just opened St Christopher's Hospice in South London, leaving St Joseph's in the East End without a doctor. She would train me at St Christopher's so that I could work part-time at St Joseph's. Thus began a thirteen year association. I spent some time training as a GP and getting some family doctor experience, but I always had sessions at St Joseph's from then on.

Some weeks after I had started this new job Dr Saunders eyed me savagely over her glasses and sniffed. 'Hm. I'm not sure what we did pray for, but it certainly wasn't you.' I remembered the Salvation Army saying 'We asked God for a garden. So he gave us some seeds.'

At first I worked in the wards at St Joseph's, under the direction of the registrar from St Christopher's. When he suddenly died, I found myself unexpectedly coping with all the medical care for ninety-six patients. We had also begun to develop the home visiting side of the Hospice's work, and I had accepted a challenge from Dr Saunders to write the first textbook on hospice care. Fortunately I had boundless energy in those days, though at times it proved uncomfortable for those who worked with me. One day Dr Saunders stopped on the stairs so I bumped into her from behind. She towered over me and with a look that sought my soul she snorted 'You're Tigger. Too bouncy by half.'

3

SISTER BRIDGET

None of this work would have been possible without the foundation laid by one of Ireland's greatest gifts to these Anglo-Saxon shores, the venerable and voluble, the holy and wily, Sister Bridget O'Gorman. I remain in her debt, with a mixture of awe and exasperation, love and reverence. Sister Bridget had not just kissed the Blarney Stone, but had bitten a piece off. When nursing, she was tender; when chatty, she was enormously entertaining; when roused, she flashed like a thunder cloud.

Coming from a north country protestant background, I was totally unprepared for the nuns at St Joseph's. The first time I visited as a student, the atmosphere overwhelmed me. Industrious, but quiet, cheerful and somehow *safe*, it is no wonder that it has the reputation for the best nursing care in East London. The nuns worked very hard with no job too dirty or menial. Their motto 'Caritas Christi urget nos' was spot on – it means 'The love of Christ leaves us no choice'. And this was the motive force that made Sister Bridget unstoppable.

When I first began to work at St Joseph's I had to adjust to a great deal. 'Sister, how can you gabble those lovely prayers?', I cried. But, 'Holy Mary Muthragod prayfrusinners nowanat th' hour' vour deathamen,' said Sister, and said it at ninety miles an hour at least fifteen times a day.

'Sister,' I asked, 'What's the logic in having the Superior sort my mail before I'm allowed to open it?' But Sister's mouth tightened as if she had pulled a lace tight. I was plainly an idiot. Sympathy was all she could offer to a young doctor who talked of *logic* to Irish nuns. Didn't I know it all came from the *heart*? And Dublin?

'How will we raise the money to pay for a salary for a social worker, Sister?' Sister rolled up her eyes like an ecstatic ikon and said, 'We'll pray,' and did. And we never ran out of money. Was it because I wrote to dozens of trusts and millionaires, or was it Sister's prayers? Or both?

We had already discharged some patients from the Hospice some years before, with a weekly follow-up clinic, because once their pain was controlled they could just as easily be home again. But there were many others who, if only they could have enough support, could also have remained at home. So in 1974 I started to make regular home visiting sessions with the Hospice patients, accepting referrals direct from family doctors who wanted to keep their patients at home, but felt a need for more skilled use of pain-killers and other palliative therapy. Sister Bridget who had an administrative post in the Hospice, was released from other duties to work full-time in this new Home Care Service.

To the peril of all East London, Sister, now aged over sixty and plagued by arthritis, took driving lessons. Perceiving the tester to be a compatriot, she started out with fervent prayer and intimidated him with fierce driving. Her subsequent triumph made the whole convent anxious, but the Superior, whose faith in us seemed inexhaustible, bought Sister Bridget a peacock-blue Mini torpedo. Soon it was to be seen challenging juggernauts to do battle on the Newham Way. 'Sister, if you have to stop suddenly, you could put your eye out on that statuette of the Virgin Mary on the dashboard.' A withering look of mingled scorn and sorrow was all the reply I received.

'And why do you cross yourself and whisper something and splash Lourdes water before you start?'

'I'm praying for the protection of our Lord on the journey.'

'But wouldn't He just prefer you to drive safely? I mean all the protection in the universe won't help you if you roll this thing over, will it?'

Sister's dilated nostrils and white-knuckled grip on the

13

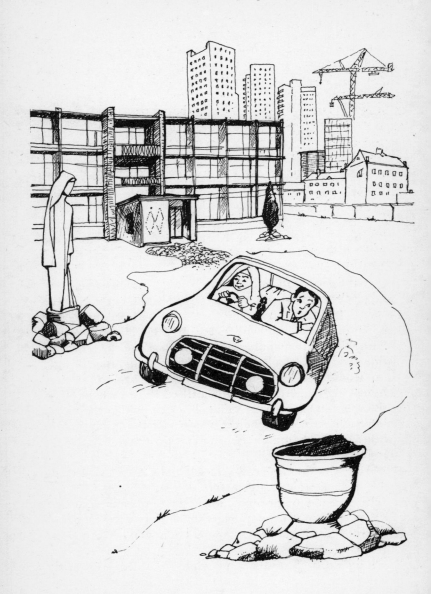

steering wheel were evidence that I had overstepped the limits of courtesy, and we swept out of St Joseph's with a roar like a fighter jet. And I was scared. Hell I was scared. And when we got back, intact, I just had to concede that some divine power had intervened, somewhere, because we were still alive and that was a palpable, verifiable, miracle.

We had visited a Mr Henry Orriss, a parks superintendent in West Ham, who was destined to be our patient for over two years. Most people were in our care about two months, but he was a fighter. Cockneys were another group for which I was totally unprepared.

'Enery Horris,' he pronounced his name, and I dutifully entered 'Mr Horace Enery' in my notes.

'Call me "Enery", doc,' he beamed and the warm-hearted Cockney magic that enthralled Dickens and Shaw had me hooked, for life. Beside him was his weary wife, looking exhausted. When I compared photos of them from that time, with how she looked, sad but fresh and healthy two years later at his funeral, I knew our care had been a success. For Henry was afflicted by a singularly nasty complication of lung cancer, which is mercifully rare, called a neuropathy. Sensation in his hands and feet was replaced by an awful burning feeling, co-ordination of his arms was lost, and his legs were totally paralysed.

At Henry's request we tried absolutely everything: pain-killers and nerve blocks, vitamins, anti-tumour drugs and steroids, radiotherapy, hydrothreapy, music therapy, physiotherapy, homoeopathic injections every day under the skin of his back for months on end, and sunflower oil. Gallons of sunflower oil, because there was a report from somwhere or other that it might help. Henry took it all without complaint. Then a neighbour read that Harry Edwards, the great spiritual healer, was in town. How about taking Henry to him? 'I don't go much on this faith-'ealing stuff, doc. Do you advise me to bovver?' So help me, I thought an outing would do him good, and there was nothing to lose, was there? Nothing out of the entire armamentarium of medicine had done Henry any good at all.

Getting Henry into the car was a real problem because he could not help himself at all. Legs and arms were just branches in the way. He needed the safety belt to hold him up. We even had a page-turner over his bed at home to make it possible for him to read a book.

Well, Henry came before Harry Edwards feeling 'a bit darft' and Harry prayed. Then he said 'Henry, stand up.' And Henry did. And what was twice as impossible, considering that a cancer deposit had destroyed a bone in Henry's shoulder, occurred when Harry Edwards said, 'Henry, raise your arms up. Right up.' The expected crunching noise never came, and the arms were as mobile as a youth's. I tell you it was completely impossible. But he did it. Boy, did I feel jealous. Seven years studying and a year of work on this one patient, and here was this guy working miracles. Medical colleagues gave smug grins of relief when I told them he was totally paralysed again two days later. But what medical treatment could have given even two days of relief to Henry?

I went through my initiation in nursing with Henry. Sister Bridget and I took turns to be on call at night, and late one evening Henry's wife came on the phone, very anxious. He was having dreadful bellyache. Please could I come? As soon as I examined him it was evident that we had failed to notice Henry getting constipated. Now he was in trouble and clearly needed an enema. It was 11 p.m. on her night off – no way could I call Sister Bridget. In the hospital a doctor can wave a lordly hand and get nurses to do the dirty work, but no such recourse was open. I would have to do it. The trouble was that I had only the haziest idea how to give an enema. I had visions of foul water squirting all over the place, so I asked for a polythene sheet to protect the carpet and bedding.

Yes, they had one. More than I bargained for in fact, because it had been used to cover a whole lawn in Henry's gardening days. So we doubled it over, spread it around and I got to work. Remember Florence Nightingale and the good old-fashioned 3-H enema. 3-H? yes, High, Hot and Hell of a lot. So we heated up two or three bags of fluid and I plunged them in. No mess so far and so I was beginning to feel more confident.

'Now, before it works I must get you onto the commode,' I said, and started lifting Henry from the bed. But there were two layers of polythene under us. One glided over the other with perfect friction-free motion. Slowly Henry and I, locked in close embrace, slid to the floor where we wrestled manfully. Then his enema worked. I squirmed in pools of brown fluid, heaved Henry up, crashed down again and completely ruined my suit. I drove home in underpants, but Henry slept like a babe.

Family and friends rallied round him in a way that I learnt to expect in East London. Henry's son took to sleeping on the floor beside his father so that Mrs Orriss could get some sleep. He postponed his wedding in order to perform this service, little guessing that he would have to wait two and a half years! To the young lady's credit, she waited. That's certainly one way of finding out if you've chosen the right mate!

————

Every day was an adventure. We never knew what we would be called on to do next. That was what made this home care endlessly fascinating. We found that, while tasks could be classified into medical or nursing, once one of us was in the house in the dead of night, we had to cover all needs. So Sister Bridget found herself taking more and more decisions with our limited range of drugs as she herself learnt to use them, and I found myself landed with all sorts of 'non-medical' jobs.

Like the night I was called to a lady who couldn't pass urine. She needed a tube put in. Now medical students all learn to put them into men, but male medics can easily get through their training without ever learning how to put in a female 'catheter', as it is called. Either I had to get one into this lady, or she would have to go to the hospital, which would be a shame. So I sorted through the anatomy books in my sleepy brain and had a try.

The room was ill-lit from above her head. No matter what position I got into, the vital bit of her was in shadow. I groped helplessly. Periodically she caught her breath suddenly, and jumped. I sweated with embarrassment and effort. But eventually I did it. Practically on my head, with her daughter holding a mirror, but I did it. I dirtied several catheters and had to discard them in the effort.

And there was Mr Peachey. When I first called, at the request of Hackney Social Services, I discovered a helpless old man too weak to lift himself out of bed. So the bed was wet, and he was very hungry. In fact it was three days since anyone had seen him, so three days since he had received any food. Nevertheless, he refused to go to the Hospice or any other hospital, saying that if he could just have some food, he would be all right.

'Well, okay, what would you like?' I asked, thinking vaguely of heating a can of beans.

'Boiled fish please, mate,' he said firmly. So what was there to do? I went out and bought some fish, boiled it to his instructions and fed it to him later.

Mr Peachey didn't perk up very much, so once he trusted us, Sister broached the idea of coming to the Hospice again. Reluctantly he agreed, and arrived very dejected. When he found that, with regular food, he didn't just die but felt much stronger, he told us about a special talent he had – playing the dulcimer. We brought it from his home, a magnificent instrument that his father had made half a century before. He tuned up, practised the hammers a bit and gave a recital of which I still have a recording. Mr Peachey became the life and soul of the ward. He told us that many years before he had even given a performance by royal command for the Queen Mother, because the fame of his playing had spread, and had featured on Eamonn Andrews' TV show.

Of course, once you accept the principle that anything goes, that whatever service people need, if it is humanly possible you will do it, you find yourself doing all sorts of things. Twice I have had a patient's weeping wife open the door to me and say,

18

'Oh thank God you've arrived – he's just had such terrible diarrhoea.' I would go in with a sinking feeling, and there he would be, covered in it, and reeking. And there she was, a sobbing heap. And there I was, and no one else. Change the bed, clean the carpet, wash the patient and bang goes an hour and a half. Talking of washing people reminds me of Winston White. Mr White was one of those very black West Indians landed with the incongruous surname of his great-great-grandfather's slave-owner. He lived alone in Hackney. It was Sister's day off, and too late in the day to ask for a district nurse to visit.

Mr White was being sullen and uncooperative. He preferred not to be examined. I decided to play for time and let him talk. At last it came out that the reason for his reluctance was that, having been too weak to get in the bath for a fortnight, he was ashamed of being smelly. So, of course I just had to bath him there and then. While the bath water heated up I popped out to the shops for some shampoo. One caught my eye that showed a glossy Afro hairdo on the container. It turned out to be a curious gluey stuff that turned the whole bath black, but it certainly worked wonders on Winston White.

Naturally the principle of overlapping roles affected other members of the team. Later when we had a social worker, for instance, she went one day to sort out a family who were making each other miserable because they couldn't communicate with one another. But on arrival she found the patient vomiting. Now you can't do a lot about family dynamics when one of them is throwing up. Being a member of our team, of course she knew exactly what to ask. The commonest reason for vomiting in a patient with terminal cancer is constipation, so she asked when he last had his bowels moved. 'Two weeks ago' was the reply. So she put in two bisacodyl suppositories and left, and that was the social worker's visit.

But I'm jumping ahead again. Sister Bridget was all the team I had at first. By the time she retired – retired, I might say,

19

to become a ward sister – the ground work was all done. Respect had been won from dozens of doctors all over the East End, and a quality of service initiated that set the standard for the next decade. Patients were being referred to us thick and fast so that we had to limit the area we served to six London boroughs and later to four. And when she went, Sister Bridget had to be replaced by six nurses.

'Would you ever,' she said to me one day. 'I went to see Mr Laffer yesterday with some blankets because I saw the hot-water bottle burns on his legs, so I guessed he must be cold, but I knew he'd be too proud to accept money. And you know that mental woman they have in the back room? Well, didn't herself come rushing out at me growling like a bull terrier and grabbed hold of my crucifix and, Lord, she had me nearly choked with it. 'Twas schizophrenia she had, they said; but if you ask me she's possessed, the poor woman.'

'So much for the crucifix protecting you,' I grumbled.

'May the Lord forgive you,' Sister gave me a withering look. 'Sure and you could do worse than wear one yourself, doctor. All she needed was a bit of pallavering. Then I made her say the Hail Mary.'

I think there were days when, in despair, the whole convent just backed away and prayed for me.

4

THE TEAM GROWS

Before Sister left, two more nurses joined us. Harriet Copperman and Clare Taylor. They were totally devoted. As the years went by and the team grew, Harriet became the nursing director. Often horrified by my madcap schemes, always pessimistic, fussing like an anxious Jewish mother, Harriet was the perfect balance for me. She had a full measure of that tantalising quality – intuition. The phone rang: 'Oh, that'll be Mr so-and-so,' said Harriet, and she was nearly always right. She could always sniff out a patient who wasn't being truthful. But if complimented on it she would just say, 'I should be so lucky,' and shrugged it off. Now Harriet has a book on the market – *Dying at Home*[1] – and is the most experienced nurse in the world in this field.

Clare was a Quaker: quiet, strong and cheerful, whatever happened. Together we all started each day with a period of silence and prayer at 8 a.m. Then at lunch time we tried to return to the hospice to eat together, followed by a further quiet time. I illuminated calligraphic texts, Harriet wove a tapestry, Clare embroidered and Sister did her spiritual reading. These spaces made the huge efforts possible. For in those days each of us was on call two nights a week in addition to the five working days.

Then two more nuns completed a district nurse training course and joined us: Sister Serena who eventually took over from Harriet as the nursing director, and Sister Hilda, a blossoming, motherly, extrovert farm girl with broad acres of common sense. Sister Serena's love of prayer and retirement made it difficult for her to crash into gear and tear away with the enthusiasm of the team at first. But it led in the end to something of much more importance. As the team grew, so did the potential for friction between all the strong personalities. It was then, searching for a deeper anchor, that we asked the Russian Archbishop, Father Anthony Bloom, to direct us in prayer, and it was to Sister Serena that the team naturally turned for leadership in this.

Two more nurses came, with each of the five health districts around us giving salaries. A succession of junior doctors joined us. At last Cancer Relief came to our aid to pay for these additions, and for a social worker who opened a new dimension for us. At last we could give family care the attention we wanted to, and could initiate a proper bereavement service.

We moulded into a wonderfully close team. Disasters hit us, and we quarreled at times, but every year the number of patients we cared for increased. Every year a higher proportion of patients were enabled to die at home. Every year the demands on our time for teaching increased.

They were a wonderful crowd. In time sixteen people worked on the team, looking after more than 100 patients at home at any one time – over 450 a year. Without deeply supportive teamwork and mutual forgiveness, such work could never have been done.

That memorable Christmas Eve night in 1976, for instance. We had had a rollicking party with piles of food. The guitar and harmonica came out as two nurses got us singing. Sister Hilda felt moved by the spirit to teach us an Irish reel in high-kicking style with much whooping. Then the phone began ringing. Sister Hilda was on call, so she set off to visit people who had phoned in with problems.

Shortly after she left, a patient who had just come on our books rang to say that he was bleeding. Cancers don't often do this, but they can occasionally cause problems. I thought I might need help, so a nurse came with me. We were still at his house at midnight, when another nurse contacted me by 'phone with a question. 'But you're not on call tonight, Clare,' I said. 'No, but Sister got three calls at once, so she rang me at home and I'm here now.'

All of us eventually got to bed except Sister Hilda who heaved a sigh of relief as she finally left a patient's house in East Ham. Then her bleeper uttered its jarring demand and she dashed back to the phone. Just a few streets away another patient had had a bleed – in two years we only had two, and they were both that night. The result was that, less than ten minutes after being phoned, the nurse arrived breathlessly on the doorstep, just after 4 a.m. on Christmas morning. The door opened and a man said, 'You were too long. He's dead.'

We gave Sister a day off to recover.

Indeed, there was a night when a nurse, the social worker and I were all at a patient's house together because a family crisis blew up when the patient took an overdose. She awoke cheerfully the next morning saying that all she had wanted was a good sleep.

I remember a staff meeting when the social worker said to me, 'Look, Richard, you've increased this patient's morphine dose three times this week, and he's still in pain. I don't think drugs are going to be the answer to that pain. Until he and his wife stop playing games, each pretending to the other that they don't know what's wrong with him, we're not going to scrape either of them off the ceiling. But, yesterday when I went to try to get them talking, he was so sleepy because your wretched morphine dose was so high, that I couldn't get any meaningful communication going. Can't you lower the drugs and give me a chance, or we'll never get his pain controlled!'

And of course I did, and of course she was right.

Now that's teamwork, and I would never want to work in any other way, having once experienced it.

Notes

1. Harriet Copperman, *Dying at Home*. Chichester, John Wiley, 1983.

5

CARE OF DYING COCKNEYS

Many elderly people are not at all horrified by the prospect of death.

An old and tired widow, Mrs McPringle, was brought to St Joseph's from a dingy flat down by the docks. I woke her up after her first night in the Hospice. She peeped over the bedclothes at me with wondering eyes, looking at my white coat, the white sheets and the white uniforms of the nursing nuns. With breathless delight she asked me, 'Am I in 'eaven?'

Another lady in the ward heard me telling a group of visiting students that our best antidepressant was a window bed – the windows go down to the floor, so a patient in bed can see out into the street and enjoy all the fights, fire engines, murders and the life of East London that he or she's always enjoyed. The following week I had another group of visitors and the patient who had overheard me, brightened up and cackled, 'Hello, I'm in the antidepressant bed.'

Cockney humour is so mercurial, barbed and uproarious. As you may know, the definition of a Cockney is someone born within the sound of Bow Bells (on a very quiet Sunday morning with the wind blowing East). Over the years we have cared for a number of distinguished Cockneys. Without one particular gentleman there might have been no more Cockneys, because he was the carpenter who rehung Bow Bells after they had been bombed in the war. Then the foreman of the Whitechapel Bell Foundry, where the bells were cast, came to us. The lady who ran the canteen from Billingsgate fish market until she was obliged to retire at seventy-five, due to weakness caused by her cancer, also died in our care. She was most resentful at being retired because the work had kept her happy. The gentleman who made the cut-glass windows for the QE II liner – cutting the beautiful patterns freehand – was another of our patients, as was a former member of West Ham United football team, also a man who had been a sorter on the Great Train Robbery train, a lady who had been cook to the Dukes of Devonshire, the Reverend Mother of Providence Row – the famous hostel for the destitute in Spitalfields, and a driver of the LMS 'Master Cutler' Pullman, as well as several stall holders on the renowned Petticoat Lane.

They're a tough, gritty, witty people. After all, look what they've been through. One home in five around here was devastated in the war. An old gentleman told me how, after a night of terrifying bombing, a German plane in difficulties crash-landed in Bethnal Green. As the pilot, who thought he was safe, climbed dazed from the cockpit, he saw a great crowd of angry East Londoners running towards him, bent on revenge. He ran like mad up the street and shinned up a lamppost. From the top he waved desperately at the crowd crying, 'Nein! Me not bomber. Me fighter-pilot!' He was rescued by a copper.

There was our Mrs Peabody who had amazed everyone in the hospital by refusing to accept her paralysis. Cancer had destroyed part of her spine and paralysed her legs. She disconcerted the nurses in the well-ordered ward at the Middlesex Hospital by dragging herself around with her elbows. Then, contrary to all expectations, she started to crawl. It should not have been possible. She began to pull herself up on the bed end, and as soon as she could wedge herself into a standing position, she announced that she was going home. Everyone protested that she could never cope, but she was adamant. So they called me. I found a rasping defiant woman with bristling red hair and a row of broken teeth – broken by her husband before he left her, so I heard. But I understand she had the consolation of knowing that she broke even more of his.

At home, still contrary to all medical prediction, she

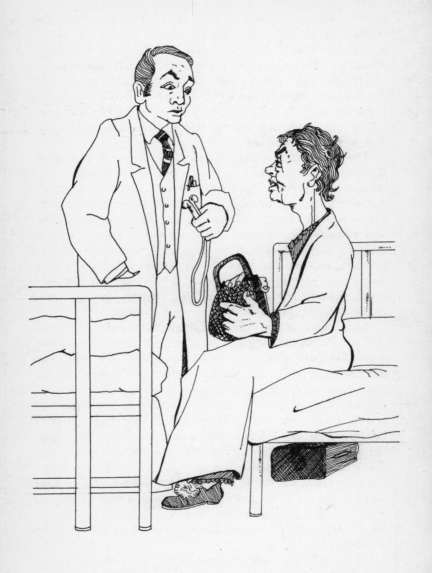

persevered with standing; then painfully, with walking with a frame. I gave her a lot of morphine, but there was no hope of totally relieving pain when she threw herself hammer and tongs into the housework. At Christmas Mrs Peabody went so far as to throw a party. A number of friends were invited, and when we arrived she came daringly to the door, in an evening gown, head held high, *unsupported*.

As if fate hadn't clobbered her enough, the cancer then spread to her brain, which produced a stroke that paralysed her down one side. Once again she was bed-bound, and extremely angry about it. The cancer continued to grow – it was evident that she would soon die. But she even did that in character, exactly as she would have wished. No gradual crushing decline for her. She had an almighty fit, and went out – BANG!

Another lady had a death rattle a few hours before her demise. (This crackly breathing in the chest is due to a failing heart which often precedes death and seldom causes the patient any distress.) It in no way marred her determination to fight; Harriet found her eating chips and reading *Woman's Own*, feebly supported on a wiry elbow.

And there was Mrs Martha Stepney, who had three great-grandchildren, all born on the same night. She waited to hear about each one, and when the third call came through with good news, she relaxed with great satisfaction and peacefully died shortly afterwards.

One lady with cancer in her spine which was arrested for two years by treatment, decided to redecorate her flat once we had controlled the pain. This she did, from her wheelchair. The same dose of morphine kept the pain away for well over a year with no question of addiction or need to increse the dose. In fact, as is so often the case, pain was not a problem. We had much more difficulty regulating her blood calcium level which changed unpredictably and made her feel ill.

Then there was Johnny Hoxton, aged fifteen, referred to us because he had a sarcoma – a bone cancer in his leg. The leg had been amputated, but it was thought the tumour had spread to his lung, so Johnny was referred to us. But as the months ticked by, his chest x-ray improved and he grew stronger, presumably cured. To help other people in his position he decided on a sponsored swim for Cancer Relief.

The prospect of the plucky lad struggling up and down the swimming pool with only one leg prompted many people to offer money, including our social worker, who thought £1 a length would challenge him. So off he went, pounding the water like a paddle steamer, and some forty-five lengths later, was still at it. To everyone's relief the baths closed, or he'd have bankrupted half of Newham.

So often the ability of ordinary people to face impending death with strength and detachment is underestimated. Bill Gravelly was someone who did so, and for whom I felt great respect. I first met him in a Salvation Army hostel in the City. Drink had lost him his job and broken his marriage. Now he was dying of cancer, aged only thirty-eight. It was hopeless trying to look after him in the hostel because as fast as I supplied bottles of morphine, other inmates stole them. So Mr Gravelly came into the Hospice at an earlier stage than was usual, and lived there for several months. He said that, as he hadn't made very good use of his life, he hoped he would at least be useful when dead, and so would we please ensure that his body was used to teach medical students?

This was arranged – when Mr Gravelly died, a demonstration autopsy was performed at the London Hospital. But in life Mr Gravelly was by no means as useless as he seemed to think. In the Hospice he gave up the drink and became a most encouraging listener and befriender of other patients who were weaker, and was to be seen sitting quietly at the bedside of many dying men. 'I was such a nice young man, I don't know what happened to my life,' he said to me. And he told the chaplain that he wanted to use every moment that he had left in serving the other patients in order to make amends, to some extent, for his wasted years. Even when he had become extremely weak he still kept this up to the last possible moment.

At the same time we had a patient coming to the Home Care clinic, who was its life and soul. Mrs Amy Wickers had an imposing presence, with a halo of silver hair and a shining smile. 'Queen Motherly' just about sums her up.

Mrs Wickers had a colostomy. (A bowel cancer or other blockage is bypassed, so the bowels discharge themselves into a bag attached to an opening made in the abdomen.) Considering her age, she had adjusted well to this operation and used to encourage others in the same plight. She had received me graciously at home, serving tea in lovely china teacups, but had complained of feeling lonely, so of course I invited her to our clinic.

It was no ordinary clinic. Once the tea flowed and everyone got to chatting, anything could happen. Sing-songs were frequent: *Die-zee, Die-zee, give me your arnswer do.* I called it our weekly knees-up. Mrs Wickers seized the spirit of the occasion and used to tell visitors a little story. The most shattering occasion came when the victim was a visiting Japanese professor. He had to put out his hand and Mrs Wickers put three matches on it. Her mouth close to his ear, she told him with a conspiratorial whisper that these represented three old ladies who were lost in Shoreditch and urgently needed the lavatory. The room fell quiet as we all watched the unsuspecting Japanese doctor anxiously.

'Ah, so,' he whispered back encouragingly.

Well, the old ladies had various adventures and the matches moved around his hand. Then they met a policeman who directed them to their goal and two of them were ok, but the third misunderstood him and took the wrong turning. Anxiety mounted as her need became more urgent. In fact she got desperate. Whereupon, unbeknown to our Japanese guest, Mrs Wickers had a damp sponge concealed in her hand 'And then, SHE DONE IT!' and warm wet fluid filled his hand.

A hoot of raucous mirth from Mrs Wickers rent the air and our friend from the Far East sat stunned for a moment. He's the only Japanese I've ever seen with an expression on his face. Then he uttered an anguished roar and ran out of the room. I

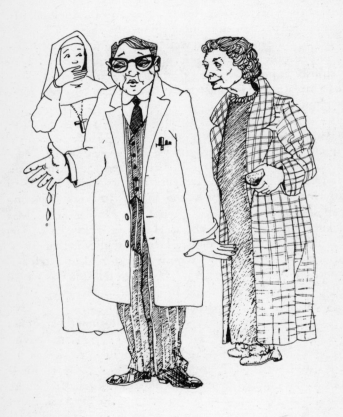

thought Anglo–Nippon relations would hit an all-time low, but that wasn't the end of the story. A few moments later he returned with a pack of cards and got his own back by confounding her and everyone else with a series of deft conjuring tricks.

Dr Kashiwagi was his name and on his return to Japan he wrote a book about his experiences in England, and opened the first hospice in that country. It was my privilege to visit it a few years ago, and magnificent work it's doing.

───────

However much fun the clinic was, though, the really deeply enjoyable part of the work was home visiting. Often in the dirtiest block of flats, with urine-smelling stairs and graffiti-covered walls, one would be welcomed over the threshold of spotless homes with polished furniture. Often there would be rather bizarre decor – orange curtains on pink walls, huge-patterned jazzy wallpaper and coffee tables rendered useless by fuzzy coverings like a ballet dancer's tutu. One family had black flocked wallpaper with yellow paint, so the place looked like the womb of an overgrown wasp, and I remember another household all fitted out with bits of boats, including a ship's wheel in the door. It gave me a tremendous sense of privilege, as evening fell, to look up at the lighted windows of a tower block and know that there was a welcome for me in several homes. Anywhere in the East End I knew the same Cockney cheer would greet me, would buy me a drink in any pub from Tower Bridge to Manor Park, and would come to our aid if the service was threatened.

When I sat listening to an old couple in their kitchen in Ronan Point, in Canning Town, I reflected on the mentality that built these tower blocks. That kitchen was one of the ones that, only a few years before, had fallen off in a gas explosion. The disaster left several people dead and Newham Council with red faces. So it should. The length and breadth of East London is a forest of these hideous towers. I have seen a young mother, from the twenty-second floor, debating with herself whether to abandon the baby or the shopping at the bottom when she came back to find the lift broken, again. She couldn't carry up both and it was a case of which was more likely to be there when she got back.

Close-knit communities were bulldozed to put up these icy fingers where people could be warehoused comfortably enough to keep them quiet. And who did it to them? Only someone who held the workers in utter contempt could promise them housing and then dump them in these isolating 'rent-slabs' as John Betjeman called them. If ever a people were *used* it was these East Enders. Whether by the old capitalist aristocrat landlords, or by the new socialist aristocrats, they have been walked over in someone else's scramble for power. But 2000 years of exploitation have not suppressed the Cockney sparkle one whit.

Take Mr Worple, for example. William Worple was a master of the Cockney rhyming slang. Until I acquired a basic vocabulary in this particular lingo, I was often perplexed. 'You can send that nurse arahnd 'ere again anytime, mate,' he said. 'Is she anybody's trouble yet? [trouble and strife = wife] Cor, lovely pair of Bristols. [You'll have to guess that one.] Don't you think so Doc?' It was he who persuaded me to try a bit of jellied eel – the local delicacy. I could relish them more if they didn't come from the Thames mud at Gallions Reach and Barking Creek – where the North London outfall sewer disgorges into the River. Mr Worple's flat always reeked with the smoke of some acrid old shag tobacco that he rolled into lip-hangers. He always wore his flat cap – even in bed – and when he died and the nurse laid him out, his daughter respectfully placed it back on his head, 'Cos 'e just don't look right wivvaht it.' Mr Worple had nearly died long before his time, because he kept falling asleep, dropping his fag and setting the bedclothes on fire. One day the nurse had been driving past and something in her mind said, 'Pop in and see Willie'. So she did, and was just in time to stifle the flames with the bedspread. One minute later and he'd have been cremated prematurely.

6

HOSPICE CARE IS FAMILY CARE

I had a thousand favourite patients, but my very favourite was Mrs Shadwell, Ellen Shadwell, a mountain of a woman. She was dreadfully nervous, so the least disturbance made her jump and ripple like a wobbly jelly. Her cancer was enormous – a lump like a rugby ball in her abdomen – but she seemed to have a truce with it. They lived together for five more years after she was referred to us for supposedly terminal care. In fact, Mrs Shadwell came near to death several times. On one occasion, with pneumonia, she came into the hospice. Her husband was also admitted because she had been looking after him. He sat beside her bed leaning on his stick, and Mrs Shadwell tenderly bade him farewell. She told everyone which belongings were to be whose and where she wanted to be buried. Goodbyes were said with many tears and jelly wobbles. Then she recovered.

She seemed to attract misfortune. One afternoon two thugs came to her door saying they had come to fix the taps. Once inside they robbed her. It was three days before she got her voice back. Since they were already poor, that left them with hardly anything.

Mrs Shadwell had a colostomy which gave her endless trouble. The biggest problem was her enormous pendulous abdomen. To find the colostomy at all, to stick the bags over it, she had to stand in front of a mirror. But as often as not, she hated it so much that she looked away, shut her eyes and slapped the bag vaguely where the hole was. So she often missed it, and it leaked, and that demoralised her more. Every time I visited she asked if I could smell it. The colostomy made her life a misery of continual embarrassment.

It so happened that, at the same time, we were looking after another lady, Miss Quirk. She also had a colostomy, which she approached rather differently. Miss Quirk was one of those rather bowel-orientated old ladies, and the best thing anyone ever did for her was to bring it round the front.

'My little man,' she called it, or sometimes just 'Charlie'. We were requested not to visit before 10 a.m. because that was Charlie's bath-time. In the living room she had rows of different potions and lotions and powders and creams for the morning ritual of tending Charlie. She pampered it, patted it and talked to it (Well, if it works for houseplants, why not a colostomy?) 'My little man misbehaved this morning,' she said staring severely into her lap one day. Clearly Charlie was in disgrace, in bad odour as they say, for the day.

So we did the obvious. We invited Mrs Shadwell and Miss Quirk to the same clinic and put them together. They talked colostomy for an hour – quite an animated conversation. ('My little man likes olive oil, does yours?') And Mrs Shadwell's whole attitude changed. She started to tend her colostomy much better. She cheered up enormously and found a new zest in life.

Her funeral was a shambles. I arrived a bit late – the people were already in the crematorium chapel and the priest was intoning the beginning of the service, so I slipped round to the side door where the undertaker was waiting. Is that Mrs Shadwell's funeral?,' I whispered. 'No, we've just brought Mrs Allen,' he replied..I peeped in. 'But those are all Mrs Shadwell's relatives!' I said. 'Who the hell have you got in the coffin?'

———

Actually, some of the East End undertakers are among the most splendid people I've ever met, providing a real service, loving care and bereavement counselling. The Pearces, the Cribbs, the Selbys and several other families do a great work of mercy. Some of them have been in the business for several generations.

Mr Hitchcock told me how his beautiful cut-glass horse-drawn hearse came to grief during the war. They were proceeding decorously down Green Street when a flying bomb demolished a house. The horse took fright and set off at a gallop with the cortège running desperately behind, trying to deflect it by waving their top hats before they reached the bend in the road. By now the hearse had gathered momentum and nothing would stop it. With a ghastly splintering the whole lot disappeared through a shop window. He didn't say where the corpse went.

Cockneys like a massive display of flowers, all over the hearse, perhaps crowned by a white cushion of flower-heads, or big letters spelling 'MUM' in flowers. One of the best displays I've ever seen accompanied Mrs Betty Coster, a Hackney publican, to her last resting place. The cortège moved at walking pace away from the 'Crown of India' preceded by old Mr Pearce, the senior undertaker of the area. In a magnificent black silk topper, with a sorrowful blood-hound face, moulded by sixty years of dolefulness and solemnity, he led them with a grandeur that even royalty couldn't surpass.

Mrs Coster had been a real character: The 'Crown of India' was in a rough area, where her pub was a haven of welcome and multiracial friendship. As her cancer began to weaken her, she made urgent efforts (eventually successful) to get the brewery to accept her son Terence ('Tel') as the licensee after her. Unemployment was beginning to increase, and she wanted to secure his future before she died. He was scarcely of age, but somehow he cared for her and the pub in spite of concurrent troubles: his pet dog was stabbed to death in the street and he had problems with his girlfriend. And some of the customers never knew there was trouble. Some folks just have grit.

We have kept contact with Tel Coster ever since, because he needs friends outside the immediate world of his pub – and because he was a tonic in himself to visit! It was Tel who taught me how to play video games by giving me free goes on his war games machine in the pub.

This follow-up of families is vital. Newly bereaved people can go through hell bacause the world expects them to 'get over it' in six weeks. Many still feel a desperate need to talk about the person who died, for two years or more after they have lost them. And if they start to get depressed, or to eat badly, they can get into medical difficulties which might have been prevented if someone had kept a wary eye on them.

I think of the Mayviss family of Limehouse, for instance. Mrs Mayviss was a great Cockney matriarch who kept her three teenage sons under her thumb – or so it appeared. In fact, I discovered that one was not her son at all. She had scooped him up when he had an affair with her eldest son, Tony, who was homosexual. While Mrs Mayviss lived, there was peace and seeming harmony. She was big enough to adjust to anything, but the rest of the family certainly was not. When they returned from her funeral, Tony, who was shattered by her loss, was summarily evicted from the flat, with his friend. As that was the only home he had known, the social worker reckoned that he had lost, all at once, more than most people could bear. We had an address in Finsbury where he might be, so I went round. The place was boarded up, so whoever was there was evidently squatting. I knocked, and a rather sexy dame with a cigarette holder came to the door and peered at me. 'Is Tony Mayviss staying here please?' I asked. From under the lipstick and eyeshadow a distinctly male voice made me jump. 'Oh don't be daft, doc; it's me!'

———

Mind you, it wasn't always a case of doing the duty of the relatives. Sometimes they kept us up to scratch. One family found a copy of my book *Care of the Dying* and quoted it every time Sister Hilda visited, and judged her every move by it.

'Richard, I could do without that wretched book of yours,' she said. 'Why in the name of all the saints did you write in it that nurses should be prepared to listen to all the family problems? Haven't I been there three hours and another dose coming tomorrow?'

But usually it wasn't up to us to do anything much beyond making it possible for people to support each other. Such was one aged couple we looked after in Plaistow. Both widowed and both in their eighties, Mr Duggan and Mrs Wintle had met at the Day Centre. It was love at first sight, and they were madly in love. And now Mrs Wintle was being snatched away. He could not nurse her, so she was admitted to the Hospice. Mr Duggan began a long bedside vigil. I came in one day to find them hand in hand, her semicomatose and him snoring gently. As it was evident that she would soon die, the nurses hadn't the heart to send him home for the night, so they made up a bed next to hers, pulled the curtians and pushed the beds close together. She faded away peacefully with her hand still in his.

Not all friends and relatives were quite so devoted. I found one Mrs Nickerson alone in her flat in a badly neglected state. As she had two daughters well able to look after her, this was surprising, for one of the wonderful things about Cockney country is the way families generally pull together – often much more than in the middle-class suburbs farther out of London. However, these two had certainly rejected her. They said she was altogether too demanding and they'd had enough of her. I was in a high old rage. 'All right. If you *won't* take care of your mother, I'll have to do it for you,' and we were forced to bring her into St Joseph's. Then I suppose they began to feel uneasy when they reflected on what they had done.

'Blimey! Did 'e say Mum's dyin'?' And they suddenly appeared in the hospice, desperately concerned, wearing so much make-up I thought they looked like a couple of clowns, or at least burnt-out tarts. Passionately gripping her hand, they never left her side. When she fell asleep they woke her up to let her know they were still there, and fussed around in a flurry of frills and cheap cologne.

'Ow Gawd! can't you just send 'em away?' Mrs Nickerson begged. Well, yes we could have. But they were only trying to make amends for their misdemeanours, weren't they? Somewhere under the crust was a good heart. So we tried to strike a balance that would care for all their needs. We let them in sometimes and turfed them out at others.

However, as I said, for most Cockneys family care is high on the list of priorities. I remember Mrs Askew – Florrie Askew – for instance. I don't think I ever saw her alone, seldom with less than three relatives present, and often with three generations of relatives. She was a matriarch, ruling her clan from her sick-bed. I suspect Mrs Askew had a number of little bargaining sessions with God. There was always just one more thing to live for. A trip to Lourdes was one of them. Now she couldn't die before going to pay her respects to Our Lady, could she? I mean, God wouldn't let the Virgin Mary down, would He? Then there was the birth of a grandchild, and then her daughter's wedding.

Unfortunately, Mrs Askew developed pneumonia when she was already very weak, and this was probably going to be the last straw. I told her what I had found. I explained to her that we probably could keep her alive, with an energetic physiotherapist bashing her chest and some antibiotics. But if I did that, it would only be a short time until her next chest infection so that, at best, I would only be ensuring that she took longer to die. I presumed she would prefer to be left in peace and not have the antibiotics?

Not so. As the wedding was next week, she wanted to be kept alive at all costs please. And so it was that we got her to the church on time, in a wheelchair, with the help of St John's Ambulance. She was extremely weak. Attending the ceremony utterly exhausted her. She turned a ghastly grey colour so that I thought she would die that night. Back at home, as we were lifting her back into bed, she wheezed to me while panting for breath, 'Now remember (puff puff) doc (puff puff) I have another daughter!'

She died well, a week later.

Many people come a long way during the time they are approaching death, and some overcome the hang-ups of a lifetime. There was Mr O'Shaunessy who became very depressed when he realised his time was running out. 'What was all that for?' he asked me.

'All what?'

'My life. It's been a complete waste. I've been a mess. A failure at everything I ever tried to do.'

Now, I thought, we can't have this. So I launched into a review of his life, asking about everything. Over half an hour later I was getting desperate. I was becoming obliged to agree with him. He really had been a mess – a thoroughly nasty piece of work. What could I do to help at this stage? I looked round helplessly for inspiration. Then there was a big thud behind me, and the answer burst in through the door in the form of his two little boys. The older one had spina bifida, he had a large head and was paralysed and the younger one carried him everywhere. They used the big head as a battering ram to open doors. In a volcano of giggles and rumpus they bounced on to his bed shouting, 'Daddy! Daddy!', and breathlessly re-counted some piece of news.

'Aha, caught you!' I said, 'Look, whether you deserve it or not, they still think the world of you. You still have an opportunity to help them.'

'How?'

'You can leave them with the memory of how a man can face death – with calm and courage, or moody and cowardly. It is your example that will be with them, as their own masculine model, for the rest of their lives.'

I don't know if our conversation did the trick or not, but his demeanour changed. He did indeed leave them with good memories, and made a quiet, dignified end.

When it is the child himself who is dying, the care needed is the same. We looked after several children at home. If hospital is a bad place for adults to die, how much more is that true of children? Provided the mother is given enough support, which means twenty-four hour professional cover such as St Joseph's offered, the child can feel so much more secure. In his familiar surroundings, with his own toys around him, with his friends on hand to come in and play, he could not be more at ease or better supported.

Dickie on the Isle of Dogs was a boy of four whom we met when his brain tumour induced coma. There was a danger of fits, so his mother had learnt how to put anti-convulsant drugs down a tube in his nose. If she was worried at all she was on the phone to us, and we knew that all calls from mothers in this kind of situation were to be treated urgently. Dickie's mother nursed him beautifully. While this went on, there were other developments in the family, drawing them together and healing old feuds.

One day our nurse was visiting them and she noticed Dickie's breathing changed. So she lifted him out of the cot, talking quietly, laid him in his mothers arms, and stayed around for a while. As they chatted, very peacefully he breathed less and less, and then stopped, cradled in his mother's arms. Because the nurse had stayed, it was not scary, and they laid him out together.

Attention to the family, always the whole family, is one of the key differences between the hospital and the hospice outlooks. Sister Serena, for instance, had a married couple in her care who happened to share the same birthday. As both were very tottery and could not leave the house, Sister organised a joint party for them at home. This gentleman, incidentally, experienced a vision a few weeks later. He said Jesus came to him and told him he would be joining him on June 25. That was indeed the date of his death.

Of course, when someone dies, the family goes on suffering. Some who have no relatives may need custodial care for a while. One old gentleman, Mr Gorman, had been looked after by his two mentally-handicapped sisters. Both were very short-sighted, needing to wear pebble-thick glasses, and both kept saying, 'Ooo-coo!', like a couple of dozing owls. Well, the poor man died suddenly, in the loo, with the door closed, and fell against it. Normally they moved like ponderous tortoises, but this event galvanised them. I was called and hastened to the house. The police were already putting their

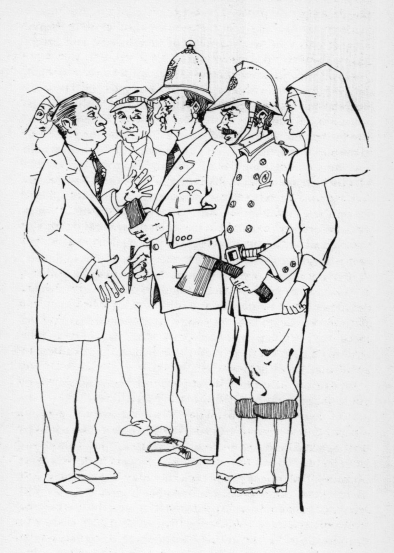

shoulders to the door when I arrived, and I was followed by a blue flashing ambulance. The sisters were leaving nothing to chance: scarcely had I got in before another siren blared outside with a firework display of blue flashes, and bright yellow fireman filled the house.

Now the negotiations began. As the ambulance was called, the ambulanceman should take the body to the Hackney Hospital mortuary as a 'BID' (Brought In Dead). But the police should report to the coroner, having already moved him by the time the ambulance came. Shouldn't they take him to the public mortuary? I don't know what the fireman would have done (cremation?), but I hit on a plan to announce that Mr Gorman's heart was still beating, so he wasn't dead, so they could all go. Then I could write a certificate in peace and call the only relevant member of the cast who was still in the wings – the undertaker. Then one of the sisters drew me aside and out tumbled all her secret anxieties. 'Doctor, he *will* be cremated, won't he? He won't be thrown in the street, or sent to Russia, or revived, or used in the cat's meat shop or anything will he?'

We had to visit those sisters regularly long after we made the funeral arrangements and disposed of Mr Gorman's clothing. His death left them quite disorientated, needing the social worker's help just to accept what had happened and the resulting changes in their lives. Their financial affairs all had to be arranged for them as well.

But most families can cope with the minimum of intervention. I like to tell the story of Mrs Churchill. This lady in her forties had come from the West Indies with four of her older children – three boys and a girl – so that they could be well-educated and gain professional qualifications. Some years later she was found to have a breast cancer. Major surgery, hormone treatment and radiotherapy had sadly failed to arrest her cancer as it spread to her liver and bones. She felt weak and ill. She knew precisely what the score was because she would tolerate no evasiveness from doctors. She had a way of tightening her lips and cross-examining them accusingly. Mrs Churchill told me she wished she could see her other children in Grenada again before she died – her passport and vaccinations were up-to-date – but there was no money to send her with.

Having relieved her pain, we made tentative inquiries as to how the the money for a flight home to Grenada might be found. One by one we met the family, and heard of her hopes for each. She said the oldest boy had turned out to be a 'bad lot' and had little to do with his mother, leaving her very concerned that the other two boys should not fall into similar ways. In particular, the younger, Spencer, was beginning to keep bad company. I told her that in her weak condition she really should have someone to look after her on the journey – a change of planes in Barbados would be involved. So she chose young Spencer to be her companion for the journey, reasoning that if she could pull him clear of London, he could work on his father's farm in moral safety. Her daughter, Sarah, and her third son, Winston, were both working, and they contributed most of the money, which was topped up by the National Society for Cancer Relief, one of the most flexible and quickest responding charities in the country.

It was a hair-raising journey. Mrs Churchill was inclined to panic before she left. The medical centre at Heathrow were just super. They arranged for her wheelchair to be fork-lifted on to the jumbo to save her the climb. All was ready and the plane about to leave when she nearly exploded. Still no sign of Spencer! He had got lost in the terminal. A manhunt ensued and British Airways had the flight delayed by thirty minutes.

We received a triumphant letter from Grenada some weeks later. She had pain again, but obviously considered it unimportant. Two weeks after that she died, just three days after seeing her second daughter married in Grenada. Then a few months later Winston turned up at the Hospice asking for work as a ward orderly, because he said it seemed a good place to be. When he moved on six months later to a training post, he told me it was the first job from which he had never taken a day off.

Now who, in this little history, was caring for whom? The

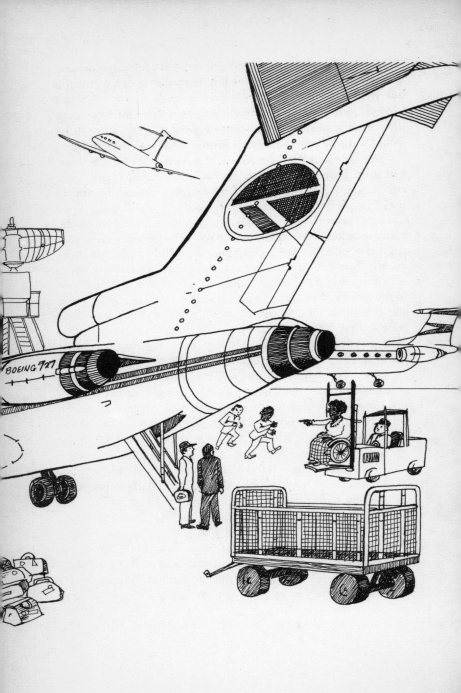

decisions were all Mrs Churchill's, every stage being discussed frankly with her. All that distinguished the patient from the rest of the team was that her role in the play was that of dying. But the team, rightly understood, includes relatives, and it should be open to the patient to take the lead if he or she wishes. Mrs Churchill certainly did, setting all the priorities.

7

PROFESSIONAL HAZARDS

Some of the corners we found ourselves in were decidedly unfunny at the time, but gave us a belly laugh to look back on.

The hazards you might expect, rarely occurred. Never was a nurse on duty at night assaulted or even threatened. We took precautions, mind you. Our area extended to Kings Cross, one of the foulest places in Europe. In some 'no-go areas' like that, a nurse on night-call was told to ask a policeman to accompany her. There was always great co-operation – in fact, there was competition. What self-respectin' copper would miss the opportunity to protect a nice young lady at 2 a.m.? Very seldom was our willingness to visit at all hours abused, but by Jove, when it was, someone got a flea in his ear. Or to put it in the inimitable vernacular of one patient:

'Blimey, mate, your nurse didn't arf give me a bollocking last night.'

'Why?'

'Well, we wanted the bed changed . . . .'

The nurses had authority to decide for themselves whether a particular call warranted a visit. In general, though, if someone were scared and rang up, they needed help.

One night when I was on duty in a rainstorm, I grabbed my bag to run from the car to the house. Dog-dirt, the bane of English towns, skidded under my foot and I landed in a heap. The patient's house had a nasty little white fence in front with spikes on top. My chin was gored and bears the scar to this day. It was sewn up by a beautiful young lady in the casualty department of the Whittington Hospital (built at the point in Highgate Hill where the great Dick Whittington did his famous about turn).

When Mr Gaynor, who had urinary problems and was too weak to stand needed to be admitted to the hospice in the middle of an ambulance strike, the roads of East London froze up completely and were nearly all blocked. Somehow we continued to function, with no accidents, and I brought Mr Gaynor into the Hospice. We were stuck in a huge traffic jam at Stratford when he announced that he couldn't wait. Quick thinking was needed. I leapt out of the car and seized a milk bottle from a doorstep. Mr Gaynor and the car seat were saved, but not without disconcerting a busload of stranded commuters in the next lane.

Our nurse, Clare, was visiting Mrs Bosham, who was in a semi-coma just before she died in a flat in Plaistow. Large numbers of relatives had arrived and were standing around the room glaring at one another. Clare tried to get first one daughter, than another to assist with the nursing care, but none was interested. 'She'll do it.' 'No, she will,' they bickered. 'But look,' said Clare, 'No one's even given this poor lady any fluid today. Her mouth is awfully dry.' Still no one volunteered, so Clare got on with things, noting that another visit would be necessary in the evening. When Clare started giving her a drink, Mrs Bosham woke up and swallowed some tea. Some of it spilt, so a change of nightdress was needed. Clare had just started doing this, when a family argument broke out about who had not been helping. Then all hell broke loose. Two men started fighting violently, glass smashed, and as Clare dived for cover a woman was thrown bodily across the room and crashed onto the display cabinet. From under the bed Clare watched in horror as people hurled each other around the room – over, around and periodically on top of, their dying mother. One gorilla of a man finally threw everyone out of the flat while his wife removed the catheter the nurse had put into the patient. Clare muttered something about calling again, and fled for her life.

But we were not often in physical danger. The emotional problems were sometimes worse. One nurse had a patient's husband fall madly in love with her. As she was laying out his wife's body he tried to grab her for a kiss. A mother whose husband had deserted her, leaving her to care for a child dying of leukaemia – most childhood leukaemias diagnosed nowadays are curable but some still are not – was desperate for support and affection. We had a conscientious junior doctor who, all unsuspecting and innocent, was very sympathetic. He was not a little shaken when she said she wished she could have a replacement baby by him. Even one of the nuns was pursued by an idolising old gentleman for a while. One cannot shake these 'transference' reactions off lightly: when a bereaved person transfers his or her love and hunger for love to the nearest kind person, it can result in very painful and embarrassing situations. (It was a cause of general mirth that, in all my thirteen years in St Joseph's, no one ever fell in love with me. 'Do you wonder, Richard?' was all the consolation the social worker offered.)

One frustrated young Arab who was dying of a muscle-wasting disease found the sexual inadequacy of his condition unbearable. Any woman in sight was grabbed. Sister Serena was his nurse, but never uttered a complaint. She had to wash him and put on new Uridoms (a sort of condom with a tube attached for a man who is incontinent). It was only after some weeks that we discovered that she had originally had an alarming little tussle. After that she gently but firmly tied him up before proceeding with the wash.

But the prize for horror stories goes to a nurse who was new on the team and didn't know how the mortuary worked. A patient had died in the hospice and a relative turned up a few days later asking to see the body. The hospice now has a pleasant private 'viewing chapel' for this purpose, with a bed and flowers. But that was still under construction when this happened. The nurse scanned the names on the big fridge, found the right body and heaved the tray out manfully. But the tray was on well-oiled rollers and shot out, knocking over the nurse who found herself grappling and grunting on the floor with the corpse. It took the relative half an hour to calm her down.

8

LETTING PEOPLE BE THEMSELVES

Everyone's experience of death is unique, so it is impossible to succeed with preconceived ideas of how people should react. To release people to be themselves meant going against common attitudes about doctors, illness and death.

Ernie Laffer was a man who made me realise how deeply ingrained some of these attitudes are. He was telling me about his biopsy in a teaching hospital. 'It was the Professor who done me autopsy, but they couldn't find nuffink.' I looked at the wrinkled abdomen on the bed before me, with so many operation scars it could have been a map of a railway marshalling yard. 'But they must have found something,' I said. 'What were all these operations for?'

'Don't ask me, mate. None of my business is it? The doctor said as how I should have it out so I did – 'e knows what 'e's doin, don't 'e?'

'Yes' but *what* did he take out?'

'Oh I dunno. Me liver was it? I'm not sure. Me liver I think.'

Such trust in my profession is humbling and not to be taken lightly.

But I have a feeling that it isn't quite right. Doctors should expect to be questioned more, and be ready to explain at some length what the treatment options are for any patient.

Hospices have made their modest contribution to bringing about this new approach. It has come in little ways. For instance, we had a team discipline that everyone readily accepted. Never did we write a patient's name – even on a little scrap of paper used as a personal memo – without putting 'Mr', 'Mrs' or 'Miss' in front of it. 'Smith, Ellen' on the hospital notes became Mrs Ellen Smith on ours. The welcome at the hospice door, the personal wardrobe for each patient, so no one took his or her clothes away, and the daily review of drugs and treatment with every patient were all little ways in which we tried to respect people's dignity.

How cautiously one must go in the face of the appalling tragedies some families have suffered! We looked after one girl in her twenties who was living with her parents. She had a little boy aged three, called Jimmy. Her husband had panicked and left her when she was found to have cancer. I don't know how she stayed sane, with the sorrow of losing her husband, the anticipated bereavement for Jimmy and fears for his future with ageing grandparents. For her parents, also, the horror must have been overwhelming. Less than ten years before, they had watched their only son die, aged fourteen, with a different cancer.

On the other hand some people need bludgeoning. Mr Forde, an aristocratic old Irishman, kept calling us out to visit him because of symptoms relating more to alcoholism than cancer.

'Tis Lord Forde on the 'phone again,' Sister Bridget said. 'Hallucinations and vomiting this time. Last time I just settled him with a glass of whiskey, may I be forgiven!' He had to be told either to stop phoning or to come into the hospice where we could regulate his imbibing. In fact, he chose the latter because he reckoned that, on balance, our 'little and often' would add up to more than the limited number of orgies he could afford. 'I'm an academiccc pherson,' he told me. 'There will be a good librarary in the hospice, I shuppose?'

We had many patients like old Miss Burdett who had winkled out of her doctor all kinds of prescriptions for an array of drugs which she took meticulously to a timetable – *her* timetable, not the doctor's. The resulting pot-pourri made pharmacological nonsense, with heart pills taken for indigestion, iron tablets to regulate her bowels and pain drugs 'for me waterworks leak', but it all *worked*. No one had any business to interfere too much, because Miss Burdett had a delicately balanced chemistry which any doctor would disturb at his peril, precipitating her into hospital if he weren't careful.

I had this conversaton with a hospice patient once:

'I think I felt stronger when I took the iron tablets, doctor.'

'I doubt if they had anything to do with it; I stopped them because I didn't think they could do you any more good.'

'Well, I think they helped.'

'Certainly they did you no harm, but I really don't want to give you any unnecessary tablets.'

'I wish you would.'

'Well, all right. Try them if you wish. Maybe I'm wrong. We'll see if you feel better in a week.'

And again:

'You're early this morning, doctor. Too early. I had my pills at 7 a.m., then a wash, then breakfast and now you.'

'Do you find it all exhausting, everything coming at once?'

'Yes. I'd love a snooze before breakfast. Couldn't I have it later?'

'Sure you can!'

And her breakfast was served at 9 a.m. ever after.

I suppose this willingness to let the patient lead and set priorities has very ancient beginnings. It goes back to the very first hospices almost 1000 years ago, which were opened as houses of hospitality for pilgrims by the Knights of St John. They cared for the sick and dying as well as for the traveller. Every morning they came into their patients' rooms and bowed, addressing them as 'My Lords the sick'.

9

DISCOVERING HOW TO USE THE DRUGS

The great breakthrough which brought the hospice movement into being was in pain control. A combination of scientific observation and good common sense led to the correct use of pain-killers like morphine in a way that is powerful and safe. But it was not only pain that needed studying. Breathlessness, nausea, dry mouth, cough, incontinence, drowsiness – all sorts of distress had to be investigated and, if possible, palliated. Drugs play an important, though limited, part in all this. We had to find, not only which drugs to use, but also the most practical way to give them. For instance, short-acting pain-killers like fortral or pethidine are of little use, because few people can cope with taking them every two hours.

Finding our way through this maze presented many challenges and some adventures. Elderly people can only cope with a small number of drugs, yet one patient produced a tray of medicines saying airily, 'I take all these.' They included several that had been prescribed for his wife, and a bottle of bubble bath.

One old Glaswegian patient found his own ideal dose of morphine. He came to the hospice from one of HM Prisons, with the pain medicine for his lung cancer in a sealed bag. He was a guest of Her Majesty for being drunk and disorderly, but the prison doctors had found that he had only a short time to live. In the ambulance he opened the medicines, and finding that one was liberally laced with gin he drained it with delight. On arrival he rather unsteadily handed me the empty bottle. I realized with horror that he had consumed about fifteen times the normal dose of morphine. I watched to

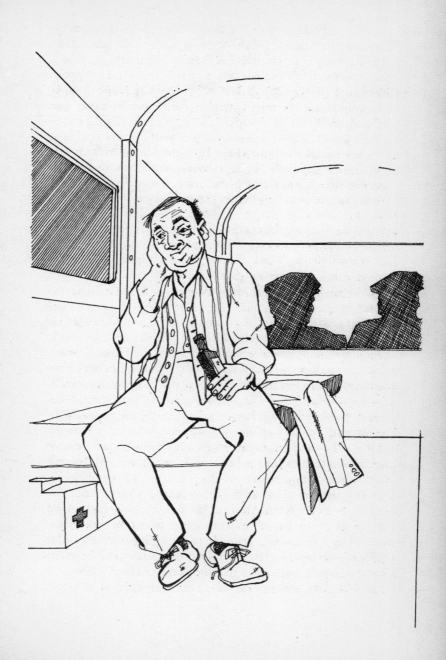

see if he would lapse into unconsciousness, but all that arose was a happy smile and 'Och, it sure got rid o' the pain, doc.'

In fact morphine is much safer than was formerly supposed. But we had to draw the line when a Mr Roscoe in Homerton ignored our advice not to drive his car. He took random swigs of his morphine mixture so that any dose might have been perilously high. Clare was his nurse, and hit on a useful tool – the mixture measure – to monitor him with. It was a piece of wood with marks on it for each day; the medicine in the bottle should only go down by a fixed amount each day. If he exceeded that, Clare warned him that he would have a day or two of pain because we wouldn't supply any more until it was due.

Most of these problems disappeared when the new slow-release morphine tablets came on the market, which needed to be taken only twice a day. The urgency of good pain control was underlined to me by one lady:

'If I don't go peaceful like,' she said. 'I'll come back and 'aunt you.'

We gradually realised that a mechanistic view of pain – as though it were just a number of electrical blips going up a cable – would not do. It has to be dealt with on four different levels – physical, mental, social and spiritual. Anxiety makes pain much more difficult to treat; the drugs just don't work as well. Tension within a family can also be manifested in the patient as pain. A troubled conscience or a feeling of pointlessness can also put pain beyond ordinary treatment. In other words the social worker and the chaplain have as important a contribution to make, even in the control of pain, as do the doctor and the nurse.

We were visiting Mr Billy Rubin who was being cared for by a very smiley wife at home. He had jaundice and severe liver pain. No matter what I gave him, the pain was unrelieved. I increased the dose several times until he was hopelessly drowsy. In the end I admitted defeat and brought him into the hospice. At once the pain vanished. Puzzled, I asked the ward sister if he really had no pain at all after admission to the hospice, even though the morphine dose had been lowered considerably. 'He had none' she replied. 'Well, except when his wife visited, then he always complained of it for a while.' Then it dawned on me that his smiley wife had a rigid, plastic smile. Obviously dreadfully tense because of the fear of him dying, she was communicating her tension and grief to her husband. And he translated it into pain. Only by breaking the vicious circle and rescuing them both had we any hope of controlling his pain.

One side effect of morphine can be a real killer, however, if the doctor isn't alert to it, and that's constipation. Mrs Samuels was referred to us half dead. She was vomiting so much that she was dehydrated; not even a sip of water stayed down. She couldn't live for more than a few days. We were told that her cancer had spread to the bowel and obstructed it. When I examined her, I just didn't believe this. I thought she was only constipated, so we got to work to relieve her. For a while enemas did no good. Then suddenly, on a Tuesday the blockage moved. One of the team found that Mrs Samuels was a lover of the ballet. She expressed such delight when a cassette of *The Nutcracker Suite* was played for her that a daring plan was instituted. The Royal Opera House provided a box for that Saturday. Mrs Samuels' son drove her to the door. The opera house staff carried her upstairs, and she was able to watch *The Sleeping Beauty* (with Harriet sitting behind with a vomit bowl at the ready, which was never needed). Merle Park and Wayne Eagling danced beautifully and were deluged with flowers at the end. After the final curtain we were manoeuvring Mrs Samuels' wheelchair out of the box when who should appear, still in full costume but those two kind-hearted dancers, to present the flowers to her. Mrs Samuels lived for another six months, resurrected by an enema.

In the same year we had three patients who died of constipation before we were able to relieve it. Their cancer was incidental to the true cause of death. We always had to be watching for constipation. One man in Stamford Hill, Mr Alec Pottager, complained to me bitterly about his constipation:

'And those things you left me didn't help either,' he said. 'I pushed two of them up but nothing happened.'

'I didn't know we left you any suppositories,' I replied, puzzled. 'Where did you get them?'

'In that little box marked St Joseph's Hospice.'

'But Mr Pottager, those were glass ampoules of an emergency pain-killer in case the nurse needed to give you an injection. You couldn't have —' I opened the emergency box. It was empty. 'You mean you pushed two of these into your . . . lie on the bed!'

And there they were, clinking ominously. We tried all manner of acrobatics, but I couldn't get them out, try as I might. So I gave him a hefty dose of laxative and let nature do the rest.

The key to proper use of drugs to bring people relief is often in the timing. How often to give them, when to start potent drug, and sometimes, even more important, when to stop one. I learnt a lot about this from Mrs Rumbelow, a lady from one of the small Caribbean islands. She had a brain tumour. When I met her she had an awful headache, vomiting all the time, and one eye was bing pushed out of place. She was becoming incoherent. New steroid drugs can make a phenomenal difference in situations like this, but in the very high doses needed, they can have most unpleasant side effects after a while, and with each increase of the dose, there are diminishing returns of benefit. Bearing this in mind, I gave a steroid to Mrs Rumbelow. The effect was dramatic. the headache and vomiting stopped, her eye returned to normal, and so did her intellect. She surmised that she must be very ill, and should prepare for death.

'I ought to think about God – soon I will be meeting Him.' She asked the nurse for a religious book. In view of her illness, and her very limited education, I thought Clare had rather overestimated her understanding when she lent her Dietrich Bonhoeffer's *Letters and Papers from Prison* – quite a theological work. But I was wrong. Mrs Rumbelow devoured it, discussing every chapter eagerly with the visiting nurses, and finishing it in three weeks. Then, in spite of the steroid drug, her nausea, headache and double vision began to reappear. It was clearly not the time to be lengthening her life so that she would die more slowly. She had had a little borrowed time and made superb use of it, but now we had reached the end. I stopped the steroid and sedated her heavily. Having used her last weeks of life for spiritual growth, she thus avoided a lot of suffering. Mrs Rumbelow was in a coma for a few days and then died in peace.

In contrast we see some poor devils who have been recklessly overtreated with last-ditch oncology drugs (drugs which deal with tumours) that make them feel awfully ill, inappropriate major surgery and exhausting hospitalisation to investigate the exact site of a cancer – merely academic because they are dying anyway. One way or another, meddlesome medical attention can turn dying into a misery if the doctors don't simply ask themselves, 'Is my proposed treatment going to improve this patient's health materially, or should I accept that he is dying and ensure that he does not suffer?' But I pass no judgement on my colleagues. These decisions can be very difficult, and sometimes we can only fall back on experience and hope our guess is right about whether or not a particular treatment would be appropriate.

10

MUCH MORE THAN DRUGS

The patient should preside over his or her own dying. We can't do it for him. We don't know his priorities. Many patients are glad to fall back into the security of a hospice, especially if they have no surviving relatives, but even more would prefer to be at home when they are dying. For most elderly folk the notion of being taken away to any kind of institution is horrific. Thus, the quality of service given by a hospice team can be measured by the proportion of their patients who die at home.

Some elderly and frail people living in flats they can no longer keep clean look like bedraggled pigeons in midwinter and rouse one's compassion. 'Oh, shouldn't she be somewhere nice, clean and warm? Can't we scoop her up and care for her?' – like Mrs Sproggett in her three pullovers with her blind smelly dog and tattered featherless budgie. But not on your life! Mrs Sproggett didn't want to be moved anywhere and was indignant at the very suggestion.

Or Mr Stocker, in his garret in Finsbury. Mr Stocker was foul-mouthed, violent and antisocial. He lived in filthy rooms lit only by candles. As there was no electricity, he illegally burned scavenged wood in an open fire to keep the place warm. Everything from the table top and the old flaking lino floor to the crockery and Billy Stocker was covered in a greasy brown film. In unfrequented corners there was a quarter of an inch of dust on everything. I used to take a newspaper to sit on when I called lest my suit be ruined.

On one occasion when I found he was not in, I conducted my examination in the more wholesome atmosphere of his betting shop across the street.

Mr Stocker had left his wife many years ago. Oddly enough, she was referred to us from another part of town about the same time as he was, and even more surprisingly, they died on the same day. We urged them to meet and forgive, but they never did. She just shuddered, and he said: 'Me wife? I'd rather 'ave a can of salmon, mate.'

Of course we wanted to get Mr Stocker into the hospice. And of course he didn't want to come.

'You do realise,' I pointed out, 'that you're getting weaker and not coping well?'

'So what?'

'Well, if you stay here, it means that one day we'll come in and find you dead on the floor. Is that how you want it?'

'Yes mate. That *is* how I want it.'

'Fine,' I said, 'as long as we understand one another, I'll certainly support you in that decision. We'll look in as often as we can and help you to stay here.'

So whether or not we agree with the patient, we obey his priorities. A confident physician will not be afraid to be guided by his patients in this way. Miss Pothecary was one who led us a dance. She chose to cope with dying by denying her plight and clinging to her proud independence. She lived alone in a dirty little flat. Her problem was intractable diarrhoea, and she was too weak to get out of the bed to the toilet. 'Never mind,' I said, 'We'll make you nice and comfortable in the hospice.'

'I'm going nowhere, young man,' was the reply.

'Well, ok perhaps we can control the diarrhoea with these capsules. Take two, three times a –'

I'm taking no drugs.' And she clamped her mouth shut to demonstrate that if I intended to force her, I'd have a tough job.

'But you can't just sit there in a pool of diarrhoea, can you?', I protested in frustration.

'And why not?'

So we had a team meeting about her. At first I was all for leaving her there till it came up to her *neck* and she finally saw sense. But in the end we said – so be it: if that's how she wants it, if dignity to her means proud independence at all costs, then we'll support her in her own way. The nurses went in twice a day to wash her and change the bedding.

———

In the care of dying people nothing less will do than total freedom to make the best end they can. Freedom from physical suffering, freedom from family and professional pressures to pretend nothing is wrong, and freedom from fear. Then, there shines through that awe-inspiring dignity and splendour that only human being passing unafraid through the gate of death can display.

Consider the story of Mary, for instance. She was a young woman of thirty-two whose bowel cancer had caused a partial blockage. We had struggled with her symptoms to get her well enough for her wedding. For her last month she was beautifully cared for in their new flat by her husband, Steve. Mary had a colostomy which Steve learned to look after. For a few weeks they were very happy. Then the inevitable occurred. The bowel blockage became total. The surgeon shook his head sadly – no further treatment could be offered. So I went to Mary and explained what had happened. Two courses were open to her. She could stay at home with Steve. To suppress the discomfort of the bowel obstruction completely I would have to give her drugs which would make her very sleepy, but I could guarantee that she would not suffer. However, because of dehydration she would only live for a few days. On the other hand, she could go into the hospital where they would undoubtedly keep her alive longer. They could give fluid through a needle in her arm, and reduce her vomiting by putting a tube down her nose and sucking her stomach empty. She may live a few weeks in this way, though I was not confident that they would control her pain. Which would she prefer?

Very solemnly Mary said she feared hospitals more than she feared death. She would prefer to stay at home and be sedated. She felt safe and happy at home with Steve by her side. So I

60

made them understand that this would be the last conversation they would be able to have together. You never get 'hardened' to this kind of situation. When Mary wept, and Steve did too, our nurse Clare wept, and then I joined in. We all sat howling round the bed. But that's all right. There is nothing unprofessional in such conduct, because it's truthful.

Then I gave Mary an injection, and she drifted into sleep. She remained like that for three days, gradually weakening, but in great peace. Then to everyone's surprise she woke up in spite of the drugs, and had one more bonus conversation with Steve before lapsing into a coma. She died the next day, cuddled in Steve's arms.

Mary did it her way. Mr Fardell did it his. Albert Fardell was an old warhorse who had been a fine leather craftsman in his prime. Both he and his wife were rather deaf, so they barked at one another. He delivered stentorian orders to her and to anyone else in the house with an iron will that never faltered. One day I took him home from our clinic tea party because the ambulance had let us down. We had to heave him out of the car and help him across a square, surrounded by council 'rent-slabs', to reach the tower block in which he lived. His pyjama trousers began to slip.

'Tie me pants up!' he ordered.

'What? his wife asked.

'Me pants! Me pants! get them fastened.'

'Oh damn you.' And she knelt before him to retie the cord, but it was not to his liking. He aimed a clout at her but she deftly evaded it, evidently being well-practised. We proceeded a few more paces when his trousers fell down completely, exposing colostomy, catheter and all to the four winds. Fascinated faces appeared in windows all round the square as he stood bottom half naked, shaking with rage and bellowing abuse at the poor woman as she hitched his trousers up again with my help.

Her health deteriorated under the strain of nursing him. It became obvious that she needed a rest. When I explained this to Albert he just reassured me that there was no such problem.

'She's coping marvellous,' he announced. Then one day she had heart failure, and I decided that he really should come into the hospice. He was adamant, however: Albert Fardell was going to die at home.

'Before or after your wife?' I ranted. Their GP went in to read the riot act later in the day, but neither he nor the district nurse made any impression on Albert's resolve. The vicar tried with some gentle little hints about the sin of selfishness. Albert, the rock, bore the onslaught with strained patience. So there was nothing for it but to apply the irresistible force. I sent in Sister Bridget, with her tongue sharpened.

He came in half an hour later. But usually there is no need to put on the pressure.

The first time we met Mrs Silverton she looked like something out of *Frankenstein*: wearing only a ragged vest, hair dishevelled, one arm swollen to gigantic size, and a big ulcer on one breast which actually did have maggots in it. Of course Sister Hilda wanted to have her admitted as an in-patient, but she could see the confused old lady was terrified. The flat smelled evil – the carpet was sticky with food and pus – but Sister quietly persevered, winning Mrs Silverton's trust in stages. She got the ulcer cleaned and covered, the old lady dressed, some food into her, and over a period of three weeks gently persuaded her that it was safe in the hospice. Of course, the first time she said 'yes', sister bundled her into the car immediately, and brought her in before she changed her mind. No doubt we could have had her certified, but no, Sister took everything at Mrs Silverton's pace, out of respect for her freedom of choice.

It isn't just leaving a well loved home that is a wrench. Sometimes, saying goodbye to a pet can be a major bereavement. So the hospice admitted dogs and other pets, now and then. One patient had a parrot which he was reluctant to part with, and when he was admitted I said I would go and bring it. It was a bad-tempered creature that sometimes swore. But it was the unpredictable and unprovoked, piercing screams it kept uttering, that made it objectionable. We were

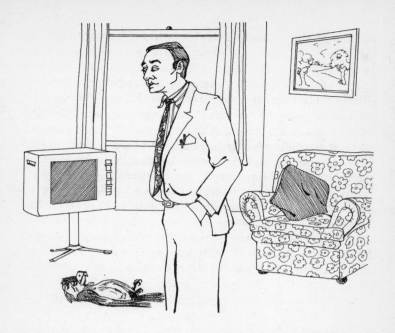

frankly dreading its presence in the hospice. The neighbours
had suffered from the bird, too. When I arrived to pick it up, I
found they had alreay seized it for vengeance, and had
strangled the brute.

We had a cheerful budgie that we used to lend to lonely
people to keep them company.

A building foreman called Mr Fritter came to the Hospice,
very breathless from a lung cancer. He hated being in bed: to
him death with dignity meant fighting to the last. He used to
drag himself to a window every day where he could watch the
men building a new wing on to the hospice, and criticise what
they were doing.

Mr Fritter asked to be spared the indignity of bed. So the
ward staff nursed him in an arm-chair. It was inconvenient,
but they did it. And unconquered, he died in his chair – a
sort of equivalent to dying with your boots on.

Mr Fitzpatrick was another who wasn't going to go

without a fight. A cancer on his foot had slowly spread up one leg over a period of twenty years without noticeably dampening his fiery energy. He was a regular and dreaded figure in the public gallery of the Islington town Hall council chamber. His raucous retorts in a thick Tipperary accent had led to his eviction on more than one occasion. Deeply immersed in local politics, he hated the cleansing department, engaged the housing department in a battle of words that lasted a decade, and wrote dark hints about the mayor to the local papers. The telephone people were all personal enemies.

His leg was a mess. I asked if he would like to have it removed? He readily agreed. When he went back to see his own doctor after the amputation, sporting his new crutches, he swung one of them at her viciously. 'Why didn't you get this old thing taken off twenty year ago, huh? Why not?' It wasn't her fault – it's just that the patient is so often not asked.

———

Given the choice, a lot of patients ask to come to the weekly tea party clinic in the hospice, for all kinds of reasons. Mrs Smith was a pious elderly lady who was grieving because of the loss of her daily Bible reading because of progressive blindness and deafness. Since I have a voice that could fill the Albert Hall, she came along eagerly every week so that I could bellow a Psalm at her. I was the only person she could hear.

Mrs Smith attributed her cancer to a kick she had received from a burglar. When I asked her if her blindness was a severe trial, she replied in a whisper, 'Yes, but it's all right. The visions above will be brighter than anything on earth.' And she shone with joy.

In contrast to her was another deaf lady, Mrs Featherstone, utterly irreverent, cursing all and sundry with a toothy guffaw. She kept a huge, moth-eaten dog to protect her that snarled and slavered at you. Even so, she was burgled and the dog done to death by some brute who must have known she was deaf.

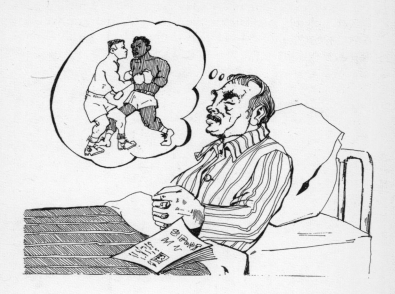

After that she lived in continuous fear, though not when she came to the clinic. Mrs Featherstone regarded me as an object of derision, and enjoyed nothing more than a friendly punch-up every time we met. Her flat was infested with vermin. The bugs didn't bother her much, but in the face of a skittering mouse she was suddenly all female, hooting from a table-top.

Yes, it was much more than diagnosis and drugs that folk needed, and they certainly appreciated our efforts. When I visited one patient, he said, 'Oh, I think I know who you are. Weren't you the doctor that visited Mr Shiner across the road last year, and sent him a card from your holiday in America?' It was a little touch I had thought nothing of, but it must have been the talk of the whole street.

Mostly it's just a case of listening to people to find out what they need. One man I met was coping with his dying by 'switching-off' and retiring into a dream world. He had been a prize fighter and just lay in bed reliving past boxing matches. I had always rather despised boxing, but when he got talking, I was completely fascinated and drawn into his dream world. After twenty minutes I suddenly realised I had actually come to ask about his appetite.

11

'TELLING'

George Deepditch described to me a conversation he had had with a radiotherapy consultant, a few months before he came to us.

'I've got an idea it's cancer,' he had said.

'No. No. No,' the consultant had insisted with evident anxiety. 'It's only a malignant tumour.'

Mr Deepditch laughed as he told me this, and added 'I'm not scared o' dying. Why should I be? I ain't never died before, 'ave I? So I don't know what it's like.' Mr Deepditch produced another of his graveyard chuckles when his daughter visited for the first time in a year. 'They think I'm dying, that's why they've come,' he said.

Clearly the doctor had more problems about death than Mr Deepditch had. This is commonly the case. Elegant professional men, accustomed to being their own masters, often find the prospect of a patient dying, or being a patient themselves, alarming. The loss of control involved with incurable illness and dying can be its most frightening aspect. Of course, if the doctor is struggling with his own fears, the patient has yet another problem to cope with.

We had one lady who, having no one to look after her at home, urgently needed hospital admission because her cancer of the nose was bleeding. But the hospital which had been treating her declined to have her back, because the ward sister refused to nurse terminal patients.

Such irrational responses from the professionals are familiar to hospice people, but none so fraught as the endless, and pointless, debate about 'Telling'. Should the patient be told he has cancer? Should we tell her she is dying? There are still large numbers of doctors who are made acutely anxious by such questions from patients, and who will avoid the subject at all costs.

What hospices find is that about a third of their patients don't want to discuss dying under any circumstances, but that a majority most certainly do. The doctor need have no rigid policy; he should just follow where the patient leads.

I had one patient who said, when asked what was wrong with her, 'It was a lump in me breast. They called it poison in the 'ospital, and I believed them and that's all I want to know.' The subject was never mentioned again.

But a more common response was that of a lady who said scornfully of her doctor, 'He didn't tell me a thing. I suppose he told my sons. I'm not silly. I do realise.' Because so many people feel cheated and underestimated in this way, we often tried to re-establish people's faith in their doctors by pointing out the doctors' own difficulties. Communication about painful topics is never easy. Most medical schools are now beginning to discuss these issues with students. But even when the doctor has made a sincere effort to explain things, it is difficult to know how much the patient understood. Certainly some people have given me most unexpected descriptions of their diagnoses.

'A malignant growth,' said Mr Fuzzle. 'It got tangled up with me thingamebobs.' And another man struggled with the words: 'I don't know what it was. Claustrophobia was it? No. No. I mean colostomy.' One lady said, 'It was a growth of some kind, they told me. I don't know much about it except that I've got it.'

Patients have displayed every possible shade in the spectrum from total denial, through suspicion, horror, anger and resignation, to complete acceptance. Here is a sample of responses I met to the question 'What did the doctor find was wrong with you?'

'I don't know. Probably cancer. I don't think about it. I say I haven't got it.'

'I know what it is, and you know, and I will not talk about it.

I don't want the others [her sisters] to know – I want no sympathy.'

'I'm a miracle, ducks, a miracle. They dug me out when I was buried by a bomb in the war, and now I've survived a cancer operation. Now I don't want anything else.' (She had discharged herself from hospital and thrown away her tablets.) 'Just let me die here, ducks, that's all I want.'

'They all framed up against me. The family, my own doctor, the 'ospital; they all knew, but they didn't tell me, see?'

'When they first told me, I defied 'em. I bought myself new socks and shoes.' This man was a cleaner in an electricity station who sat reading *The Daily Telegraph* and making wry observations on the ways of the world. He had already concluded that he had inoperable cancer when the hospital doctor told him cheerfully that he could smoke as much as he liked. His defiance continued until a few days before his death. He stayed at home, a recluse with neither friends nor family, dragging himself into his kitchen, untidy for the first time in years. He kept burning himself when he fell asleep, and dropped his cigarette. Only when totally overwhelmed by weakness did he reluctantly agree to hospice admission.

A Mrs Simpson told me she didn't know what was wrong with her. I noticed that she was dismissing the subject rather airily, so I asked what she thought it was, and she whispered, 'Cancer.' I said quietly, 'Yes, but not a nasty one.' 'It's all right, my dear,' she replied, 'I'm not frightened.'

And there were those who simply saw no problem at all in death, like Mrs Martin who, five weeks before her death, correctly predicted that she would die on St Joseph's Day; or the lady who, when I asked whether her husband were still alive, said, 'No. He passed on six year ago. 'E's over there.' I jumped and followed her pointing finger across the bedroom. On the dressing table was a little urn of ashes.

———

For many people the process of coming to terms with their dying was much helped by the willingness of the hospice staff to talk about it.

One lady who had been very demanding, protesting energetically about her weakness and demanding instant cures from her doctors, assailed me when I arrived in a hailstorm:

'Can't you bring good weather, doctor?'

'No!'

'I'm asking too much of you, aren't I?' she suddenly mused, and laughed when her husband said, 'Yes. In every way.'

When we first met Mr Murdo Craigie he was reading a book called *I Conquered Cancer*. His father-in-law had died in St Joseph's and he angrily rejected the idea of admission. 'I don't want to go into that place. I want a specialist to put me right,' and then in desperation he added, 'I'll pay!' Of course I had to tell him that a mint of money couldn't make him well. Gradually it sunk in.

Percy Becker was a man who was considerably helped by talking. His pain, from a cancer deposit in his hip, proved impossible to control. We were giving him more and more morphine with no benefit. One evening his parish priest and I arrived on the doorstep together. I was hoping to avert another sleepless night by giving him more pain-killers. However, because the priest and I were both there, Mr Becker asked about death for the first time. It became evident that, while death didn't alarm him much, he was very anxious about dying, so I probed a bit to find out just what was worrying him. It turned out that he had two fears which are both common, and both unrealistic.

The first was that he thought the cancer would in some mysterious way creep up one night and strangle him. I have been surprised to find this fear of cancer coming up into someone's throat is widespread, even in countries as different as Canada, Zimbabwe, Germany, Trinidad and Japan. My impression was that the fear plagued almost half of our patients in East London. Yet I've never seen it happen. It is very rare for a cancer to close someone's throat, and even when it does, it does so very slowly so the doctors have plenty of time to put in

70

a 'tracheotomy' breathing tube. So I told Mr Becker there was no question of his cancer choking him.

The second fear was that he might wake up in the crematorium, not really dead. I promised him that I wouldn't let the undertaker move him until his body was cold and stiff. Mr Becker was visibly relieved. Next morning his wife phoned to say he had no pain. We tailed off his morphine dose until eventually he had only aspirin. His pain remained totally controlled for months. It had been due more to anxiety than cancer. We meet this 'mental pain' all the time. Often an honest chat can lead to its relief.

When I was a young doctor doing my first hospice job, I encountered a lady who needed to face the fact that she was dying, squarely and honestly. She had been a real trial for the nurses, complaining and irritable. I listened to her and thought, 'This is ridiculous. She's just sulking, and making what little life she has left hell for herself, as well as for the nurses.' So I told her so, 'You're behaving like a sulking child, Mrs Horner.'

What a response! She was blazing angry. A complaint went up the administrative hierarchy; the nurses were outraged, and Mrs Horner refused to talk to me. But I was sure of what I had said, so I stuck to my guns. Only the psychiatrist supported me. 'She's not done anything so positive as this for weeks,' he observed. Another week passed. Every morning when I did my round she pretended to be asleep, and I ruffled her dignity by slapping her on the shoulder and giving a cheery greeting. Then one morning another lady in the ward was celebrating her eightieth birthday with great gusto. Mrs Horner's chair was facing the wall, shutting it all out.

I stuck my face round and said, 'Hi there! What a super party, isn't it?'

She looked at me and considered. Then slowly and deliberately, like one who had come to a decision, she said, 'Hm. It's nice to see you, doctor. Will you turn my chair round so I can join in, please?'

And from that day on she was a much happier person,

considerate of everyone around her.

Actually, the patients themselves are generally easy to help: the relatives present many more difficulties. So often they won't let anyone talk to the patient about his fear of death because they themselves find the subject too painful. They're actually protecting themselves, while the patient becomes terribly isolated and frightened. Nothing cuts you off from people more than false reassurance.

We had one patient who was not at all worried about dying and told me so more than once. But he had a really fierce wife. On her doorstep in Pentonville Road she had fixed me with an eyeball–to–eyeball glare and said, 'Listen 'ere: you tell 'im, and I'll thump yer.' Obviously, the one with the problems, who needed all our help, was her, not the patient, but I didn't argue. I looked at her muscles and decided discretion was the better part of valour. It was some time before she realised that he really wanted to share it with her and say goodbye properly. Many people feel wretched when someone dies having never been allowed to say goodbe, or sorry, or thank you. A silly charade is kept up, sometimes involving deceit and evasion which make a mockery of a good marriage. I have even known this to be the result of medical advice from doctors who should have known better. Occasionally, I've asked patients:

'What did the doctor find wrong with you?'

'They never told me.'

'Did you ask?'

'No.' (pause) 'Doctor, these false teeth don't fit; can I have an appointment with the dentist?'

That is one response, and should be respected. But quite another is more usual:

'Of course I want to know!', said Mrs Gordon. 'I've never been a coward. I fight.' 'Mind you,' she added, 'I don't fight with me 'usband. He's too frightened of me right fist.' (I think she threw that in to resssure me that she would co-operate with us provided it was on her terms.)

The extent to which families will go to prevent this open

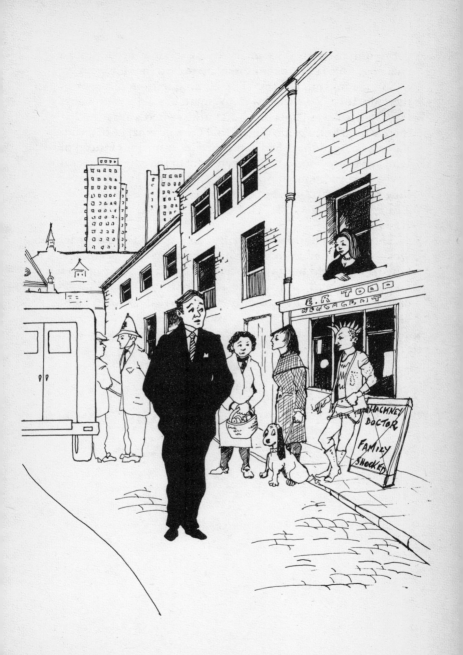

communication that so many dying people need can be amazing. One lady tried to force me to lie to her husband by asking me in front of him, 'There's no question of cancer, is there doctor?' When she was not there he told me he knew exactly what was happening, and just wanted assurance that there would be no pain. When I told his wife what he had said, she was enraged that I had confirmed his suspicions instead of lying, and threw me out. She then went to the editor of a local newspaper and poured out her anger to him. To my horror they made it a front-page scandal: 'HACKNEY DOCTOR TELLS CANCER VICTIM HE IS DYING – FAMILY ANGRY.'

The cause of her anxiety finally came out when our social worker paid a bereavement visit after the patient's death. His wife had thought his lung cancer was going to come up and out of his mouth, and wanted to spare him such a hideous death-sentence. They had only been married six weeks and had not yet established that easier communication which comes from knowing someone's habits over many years.

12

EUTHANASIA

We had a lot of trouble looking after one old Irishman in Haringay because his inexperienced young doctor had panicked and over-prescribed. At every visit she kept writing until a prescription form was full. (To reach for a prescription pad when you feel impotent is a common medical reaction.) But it gradually became evident that many of Mr O'Flaherty's symptoms were actually bizarre drug interactions. The reason was made only too clear on the day he died. His wife said, 'Oh, and doctor, you'd better take these,' and handed me a bucket yes a *bucket*, full of tablets. Because of a conversation she had with Sister Bridget later that day, I called again later in the week, only to be presented with the *other* bucket of tablets that they had kept in the bathroom. All free on the National Health of course.

Sister Bridget had given Mr O'Flaherty an injection, some hours before he died, because his pain-killers were wearing off, and he was no longer able to swallow. When she called to console his wife that afternoon she was shattered by an unexpected attack.

'You killed him. You gave him that euthanasia injection. don't say you didn't: we saw all about it on TV.'

That was back in 1973, and it was the first time the question of euthanasia had ever come to our notice. Of course Sister's injection did not shorten Mr O'Flaherty's life at all – it probably lengthened it a little if anything, by preventing exhausting and pain-wracked restlesness.

What the media debate about euthanasia has done, more than anything else, is to terrify lots of people. I have had three old ladies refuse to go into hospital simply because they were afraid that someone there would kill them. Neither has the Humanist lobby, who keep fighting for euthanasia, done anything to reassure people. The 'Exit' fiasco of the Nicholas Reed and Mark Lyons 'assisted suicides', Arthur Koestler, who was quite happy to let his healthy young wife kill herself to avoid living on after his own death, and the three Euthanasia Bills presented to Parliament which offered no safeguards at all for preventing pressure being put on old people with relatively minor ailments to do away with themselves 'voluntarily' – all these have combined to give a macabre image to the Euthanasia Society. We should steer clear of such ideas, or some day someone might creep up and hold your head under the bathwater.

If someone really is eager to die, a sensible response would not be to agree and kill them at once, but to ask why. There will always be a good reason why someone wishes they were dead. What hospices maintain is that good care will eliminate those reasons, so that the vast majority of candidates for euthanasia will change their minds if they are properly nursed.

Mrs Langton – Mabel to all her friends – died aged seventy-nine. On account of what she called her 'Arthuritus' she had spent forty of those years in hospitals, including most of her childhood, because she had dislocated hips for which treatment was not known in those days. Mabel was bedbound when I first met her, grumpy as a toad, and always in pain. I dreaded coming to her bedside on my hospice ward-round, because she always had the pain which seemed resistant to all my medications, and a host of other minor complaints: indigestion, sore mouth, cataracts in her eyes, severe itching, sore throat, sinusitis, hard bed, bad food, uncaring nurses, and so on.

'I wish I was in me box,' she used to spit out, peering balefully through thick glasses. Sometimes *I* wished she were. But I asked an eminent rheumatologist how to help her. He said to ignore the rheumatism and focus on the chronic depression. So we put her in a window bed, gave antidepress-ant drugs and searched for some occupational therapy. She admitted she had once been good at knitting.

'Mabel, in this weather I'm awfully cold in the car. I need a scarf urgently. Would you knit me one?', I asked. I found two very thick knitting needles that could be gripped by her deformed fingers, and some thick scratchy blue wool.

Mabel was very reluctant at first. She hid everthing in her locker, but I pulled it out. I went in four or five times a day to say 'Mabel, get knitting!' At first it was full of curses and dropped stitches, but gradually the standard improved. She triumphantly ran out of wool, but I bought some more. When it was five feet long she asked, 'Isn't that enough?' 'No', I replied. When it was seven feet long and right over the end of the bed, she put a row of tassels across it to prevent me demanding anything longer. So I bought more wool, and asked for another scarf for my girlfriend, who was also cold in the car.

Mabel cheered up tremendously. I no longer needed to urge her to knit. Bedjackets and blankets came off the production line, and finally an exquisite tea cosy with two matching egg cosies in tiny stitches of four different colours of wool. As my marriage to the above-mentioned girlfriend was now imminent, a beaming Mabel presented us with the cosy set as a wedding present. In fact she beamed at everyone, except when the nun in charge of her ward extracted a notorious piece of pornography from under her pillow.

A few weeks before she died, I asked Mabel if she still had pain. Her reply, after forty years of grumpiness, was astonishing:

'Oh yes, but it's no trouble.' There, finally laid aside, was the hang-up of a lifetime. Certainly it took other people's help – that's why the Almighty put more than one of us on the globe – but the great step forward was entirely her own. What if euthanasia had been legalised and she had been able to demand it for her unrelieved pain a year earlier?

We had a gentleman with severe neck pain. He said he had been in agony for three months in the hospital before he came to us, and asked the hospice doctor to put him out of his misery.

A week later he was pain-free, and eventually went home where he lived for several months. Another, Mrs Bassett, also found hospitals unable to help her. 'I felt like a leper in there,' she said. 'When I told them I had pain they said I was an old moaner and a nuisance.' Mrs Bassett was one of five people we found for a TV programme being made about euthanasia, who told the interviewer that they had longed for euthanasia until they became hospice patients, but were now glad to be alive.

Another of those five was Mrs Emmott. she had come to our regular tea party some months earlier, very depressed because her husband had recently died. She was herself weakened by cancer and the grief had caused a flare-up of her arthritis. Life was not worth living, she said. Couldn't I just finish her off, please – that euthanasia thing she'd seen them talking about on the telly?

'You mean you want me to kill you?'

'Yes,' she said, 'I do.'

'Well all right then,' I said reluctantly, 'no one would know, I suppose. Only myself and the nurse – and she won't say anything, will you, Sister?' (Sister Hilda shot me an anxious look.) 'We'll do it now, love, with an injection. Hold your arm out. Sister, pass me a syringe – no, not that one. The big one. We'll need a lot to be sure to kill her. Come on, Mrs Emmott – hold your arm out.'

But the arm was behind her back. She gave a nervous giggle (Sister Hilda was looking quite demoralised). Then Mrs Emmott said something that I will never forget: 'No, doctor. What I mean is, aren't you going to do something to help me?' What a lesson there was in her words! When aged or dying people request euthanassia, that is a desperate cry for help.

Are you cold? Are you lonely? Is your pain inadequately controlled? Never mind. I'll put all that right. I'll kill you.

What a daft response to human distress! We should be thankful none of the death brigade were around when people were struggling to conquer smallpox, cholera and TB, vagrancy and poverty in our society. Of course I don't advocate keeping people alive artificially when they are at the end of a terminal illness, but neither is it ever necessary to kill anyone. A patient who is begging to die has lousy doctors and nurses, that's all.

We knew another lady who slashed her wrists and took an overdose, to be resuscitated in Casualty, who then climbed on the parapet of Tower Bridge – to be yanked back by a copper. But once we enabled her to be at home with her four children, she decided not to do anything like that again for their sake. Families can feel awfully guilty after a suicide. If euthanasia were legal, what would the misery be like afterwards for relatives who had been hectored into consenting to the killing of their kin?

In a public debate on life after death in Hackney with two prominent humanists, our social worker concluded by asking the audience which of the disputing teams – the Jew, Muslim and Christian, or the humanists –*looked* happier. It was a good point to make in our team's case! The intellectal chatter generated by euthanasia and other humanist causes is so drab beside the fiery energy and delight that come to giver and receiver in the simple service of fellow human beings. When one is weary with arguing there is nothing left but to go back and help someone successfully confront his problems.

———

The last words shall go to a patient and two relatives of patients. Here are extracts from letters they sent to the media:
To *The Guardian*, 22 November 1976

Recently my wife was found to be suffering from a highly malignant carcinoma of the colon. After a month in hospital where palliative surgery was performed, she was given a supply of pain killing drugs and was discharged. Although these drugs controlled her pain, they had various side effects, the most serious of which was permanent nausea, making it impossible for her to keep down food.

We were fortunate in being referred to a local hospice specialising in care for the terminally ill in their own homes.

Under their skilful use of drugs her pain was controlled and so were the side effects. Her last six weeks of life were very happy ones, and she was able to achieve many things she thought she would never be able to do again. Only the last few days were spent totally in bed, and even then her mind was very alert.

It seems that many people in the medical profession and outside it, are unaware that it is possible to care for incurable patients in this way. I wonder if the percentage of people wanting voluntary euthanasia would be so high if it was generally known that the quality of life, even in advanced terminal illness, need not be unduly diminished?

S.W. BARNETT, London N4

To *The Hornsey Journal*, 1977

My husband has just died of cancer which had caused paralysis of his lower body, but at the point where it would have become unbearable for him and terrifying for me, the team from St Joseph's Hospice took over his care. At no point was he allowed to suffer. Never was I without immediate help if I telephoned. The result was that I was able to look after him to the very end, and he was never driven to express a wish to die.

The sooner this kind of service is available everywhere the better. Then euthanasia will be a meaningless idea.

Mrs M. CHRISTIE, London N19

To Granada Television, 4 August 1980

My cancer was diagnosed in November 1979 and my health deteriorated rapidly thereafter. By January of this year I was bedbound by pain and weakness, having been able to drink only water for six weeks. My wife had been told by our family doctor that I 'would die a painful death within three months'. I felt desperate, isolated and frightened and at the time I truly wished that euthanasia could have been administered. I now know that only my death is inevitable and since coming under the care of the St Joseph's Hospice home care service my pain has been relieved completely, my ability to enjoy life restored and my fears of an agonising end allayed. As you can see, I'm still alive today. My weight and strength have increased since treatment made it possible to eat normally and I feel that I'm living a full life, worth living. My wife and I have come to accept that I'm dying and we can now discuss it openly between ourselves and with the staff (of the hospice), which does much to ease our anxieties.

My experiences have served to convince me that euthanasia, even if voluntary, is fundamentally wrong and I'm now staunchly against it on religious, moral, intellectual and spiritual grounds. My wife's views have changed similarly. I'm no longer in such misery that her love for me would make her want me to be dead. And after I've gone she will not have to fear the burden of guilt which would have been upon her had she wished for my early death. None of these feelings of mine were made clear to the viewing public in your programme which did nothing to shake the accepted view of cancer as a lingering, painful death, which can be avoided only by euthanasia. This lack of clarity was brought home to me when I was stopped in the street by an inquisitor after the programme and asked 'was I for or against, after all?'

SIDNEY COHEN, London E7

13

IMMIGRANT PATIENTS

'What's your religion?' I asked one bright-eyed old lady.
'Cockney' came the reply, with not a flicker of an eyelash.
I looked up. 'Yes; salt of the earth' I said.
She smiled modestly. 'Well, yes, I suppose that's true.'

When your roots go down 2000 years and your father had the same Christian name as his father and grandfather and so on for six generations back; when three generations of your family live in one street; when you are totally satisfied with your place in society and are ready to die for the Queen, or live for your neighbours; when you have fought fires in the battle for survival during the Blitz when one house in five in East London was ruined; when you are proud of your heritage and draw lifeblood and meaning from your community, you cannot understand how the immigrant feels.

Cockneys have absorbed wave after wave of refugees from Europe for hundreds of years, but the last generation has seen an overwhelming influx of people from every continent on the planet, who share no common cultural assumptions.

Recent immigrants pose a particular problem to the medical services. There are different ways of describing pain or other physical symptoms, even if there is no language barrier. Arabs and Pakistanis have no concept of doctor or nurse to correspond with ours, and thus no idea how to use them. Different parts of the body are taboo. Some races expect doctors to make a diagnosis without even touching female patients. Concepts about the nature of disease differ. To bridge these gaps enormous goodwill is needed on both sides. Many West Indians, for instance, have had so many experiences of rejection and hostility that they genuinely fear we might come to kill the ill family member. Trust can take ages to develop.

However, Mr Green was one Jamaican who had no such problem at all. When he first found he had cancer he had been rather angry and withdrawn, but then he began to think about it. He was a merchant seaman who had taken to the oceans because he wanted adventure. It dawned on him that dying was going to be his most exciting voyage ever, so he settled back in eager anticipation. About that time a TV company asked if they could film a dying patient. My initial reaction was, 'This is a hospice, not a zoo; get to hell out of here!' But then I thought of Mr Green. He rose to the challenge with delight, though none of us realised what he had in mind.

Miles of wires, cameras and bright lights crowded into his little bedroom and an interviewer with a reaction of terror to the mention of death sidled up anxiously. Mr Green interviewed him with forthtright gusto. No, he didn't mind dying; of course not, why should he? It was natural, wasn't it? Why did you British have such problems about death? Look at the ridiculous game he had seen in the hospital when a patient died: curtains pulled round, whispering, a squeaking wheel of a trolley . . ., profound silence, then all of a sudden a breezy nurse whisked back the curtains, all cheerful and chatty and pretending nothing had happened! And look at those absurd English funerals. Everyone trying not to cry – how stupid! Everbody wants to cry, but nobody does. Most people stay away to avoid a scene and all you bury is a box. Nobody ever sees whether there's a body in it or not. Hundreds of pounds on flowers, but not one person expresses any real feelings.

Mr Green warmed to his subject. The English go on like this because, in the face of death, they are just cowards, he said with a broad smile. Every immigrant in the land must have been watching him with envy. Hitting back at these cold English people from such an indisputable position of strength. And did he enjoy it! Back home in Jamaica it was all handled much more sensibly, he told us. A funeral is a time for expressions of great community support and solidarity. Hundreds of people would attend, all in respectful best clothes. The family were encouraged to wail their protest at God or weep their sorrowful submission. The body would be visible to all, especially the children who could thus see that death is not at all terrifying, just the discarding of a husk which is obviously not Grandad himself. Afterwards, the family would be helped by hosts of relatives and neighbours until the numbness and shock had subsided.

Abrasive he may have been, but I suspect Mr Green had a lot to tell us. Not just Mr Green. This sense of family and communal unity is a great contribution our Caribbean immigrants can teach the English if they can be humble enough to learn.

—————

It is necessary for health-care workers to understand a little about foreign religions. I visited one West Indian lady for the first time while she was still in the Prince of Wales's Hospital. Because of our difficulty in establishing a trusting relationship with some black people, I was determined to get it right from the outset with Mrs Cholmondeley. I asked what her religion was.

'United Church of Cherubim and Seraphim.'

I knew what that meant: a passionately evangelical Christian group, such as are found in many West Indian communities. So I said confidently, 'Oh good. I'm a Christian too.'

The lady rolled her eyes. 'Thank God for that!', she said. 'No one else in this hospital seems to be.' Then a slight cloud passed over.

'What kind of a Christian?' Piercing eyes turned towards me. Had I been a Catholic the relationship would have perished. 'A Quaker.' She had never heard of them and looked interested.

'Are they like the Brethren?'

'Oh, more or less', I said vaguely, not entirely sure. Anyway, she let me off the hook and I examined her. When I was ready to go I offered to say a prayer with her, because I knew that she would want to begin and end all activities with an expression of the great piety she felt. She looked delighted. I glanced around. The other patients were at the end of the ward huddled round the television. The doctors and nurses were having a meeting in Sister's office. All was quiet so I knelt down, expecting to say a few words of thanksgiving – that we had met and that Mrs Cholmondeley could now come home. But she threw out her arms ecstatically and hollared:

'HALLELUJAH!!!'

I gasped and looked up. The nurses and doctors came out to see what was happening.

'Thank you, Lord', she intoned, 'for bringing me a Christian doctor at last.' The patients left the TV and gathered round to watch. I began to sweat.

'Glory be!' wept Mrs Cholmondeley and then, to universal fascination, she began to speak in tongues. Streams and streams of a foreign language, chunks of the King James Bible, miscellaneous 'hallelujahs' and 'Praise the Lords'. After about five minutes she at last paused for breath and I firmly said,

'AMEN!'

Needless to say, we got on like brother and sister after that. In fact, our Sister Serena found kindred spirits among several West Indian families because she also loved nothing more than to pray and praise.

———

Bangladeshis are some of the most difficult patients to understand.

'She got a burning, oh terrible burning, in the belly here and it come up and turn and go out down the arms and nose.'

One lovely family urged me to visit on a particular day to share their end–of–Ramadan feast. I was quite unprepared on the appointed evening for the mountains of food that this really poor family produced. As I munched through spiced meats and piles of rice I was watched by an exquisite row of infants from nought to five years old in ethnic dress. But after a while their attention drifted to the television next to me. When the whole row gasped and cried out together, I turned to see what they were watching. I was just in time to see the *Jaws* shark biting off a man's leg, and I nearly threw up the whole feast.

Several patients from both East and West Indies have wanted to return home to die. By the time they realised that death was imminent, these people were often really too weak to travel. Massive efforts by families and painstaking airlines, especially the medical centre at Heathrow, enabled them to realise their dying wishes. Several had to take supplies of drugs with them – several litres of morphine solution, for example. Somehow, customs officers never quibbled. The morphine was legal, as far as I know, but I wonder if some had more than the duty-free limit of alcohol mixed in with it!

We had real trouble with one family. The Pakistani husband had abandoned his English wife and two boys and gone back to Pakistan. Now the wife was dying. What was to become of the sons? They had always lived in England. A relative attempted to kidnap them and whisk them off to Pakistan. The prospect horrified the boys and since the Tower Hamlets social workers were on strike, there was no one to defend them. Our social worker battled to avert disaster and found a lady who knew them and would act as guardian while a solicitor made them wards of court.

An Arab patient who broke all the records for travelling was Mr Bouadja. His liver was full of cancer, filling his whole abdomen. I was dubious about his Planned visit to North Africa, but offered to find him a lift to Heathrow. 'No, not Heathrow,' he said. 'Victoria, please.' He was going by *bus*! Three days each way! He departed cheerfully. 'What present can I bring you, doctor?' he asked. 'Oh, a camel,' I laughed.

Three weeks later he reappeared triumphantly. We welcomed him to the clinic. 'Doctor,' he beamed, 'I bring you camels!' I started and looked anxiously into the garden. But he pulled out a case and produced a row of leather model ones that he had carried all the way from Africa. No sooner had Mr Bouadja settled back home than his father died, so he made the whole journey again. Whenever a family crisis arose, his son rang us up and said just two words: 'You come?' It might be Mr Bouadja having a severe pain (I never understood why, but since it always responded to simple treatment, I didn't fuss), or it might be the defective plumbing in the flat, deluging them with sewage again, or a strange epidemic rash afflicting the whole family (lice). They certainly appreciated the British welfare system. The first time our social worker visited Mr Bouadja he welcomed her warmly. 'Come in! You bring house?'

Harriet and I were once treated to a slap-up meal by a family from Shanghai who ran a Chinese restaurant. Harriet felt sick, so I ate hers as well. I think our communication difficulties were at their worst with Chinese families. Older members spoke not a word of English, and some of their customs shocked us. For example, when Mr Deng was dying, his family insisted, inspite of all our pleading to the contrary, that he should be sent into hospital. When the ambulance arrived, his wife lunged at him with a pair of scissors and angrily cut off all his buttons. Quite what this signified I never could discover, but his response was a look of utter dejection and despair.

———

Patterns of grieving differ enormously too. If an Englishman screams and throws himself about with grief, he's probably at psychiatric risk. If a Greek does *not* do these things, he's probably ill.

I once went to write the death certificate of an Italian patient. When I reached the street, I realised that I had forgotten the house number. I need not have worried, as I had only to get out of the car and listen. It was No. 15, as wails and groans revealed. People need to grieve in their own way. I remember a horrified nun at St Joseph's trying to shush seventeen members of an old Italian grandfather's family who gradually gathered round his bed during his last night. They waited, tense and poised, as his breathing failed. Sister knelt beside him, repeating the prayers for the dying. She felt his pulse: it flickered to a stop. Then she said, 'He's gone now,' whereupon the entire company started howling and two disconsolate women hurled themselves across his chest whooping in paroxysms of remorse. The corpse took a mighty gasping breath and uttered a final satisfied groan.

It can all go terribly wrong in England's green and pleasant land of showers. One of our Greek families went through the time-honoured ritual. Inconsolable wailing at the cemetery was accompanied by people abondoning themselves to their grief. One lady beat the ground with her fists. In Cyprus she could have shaken off the dust, but in London it was a porridge of mud. The eldest son wept unashamedly and declared he should be buried too, attempting to leap into the grave while others restrained him, as it is their traditional duty to do. But again, the mud reduced the gesture to a fiasco, while the staunch immobility of our social worker and the pin-striped undertaker contrasted ridiculously with the florid expressions of grief around them, so that in the end everyone looked funny.

––––––––

The problems of the immigrant were well illustrated by the adventures of Culdip, an Indian junior doctor who joined our team. He kept colliding with nurses at the swing doors, because each expected to go through first. He was dismayed to find himself berated for letting a nurse carry things for him.

'Culdip,' I remonstrated. 'Can't you see Sister Hilda struggling with that commode? Help her!'

'I have *never* carried anything for a woman,' he protested.

'Then you can bloody well start now. You're not a maharajah here.'

Poor Culdip went to see a patient who was having a lot of pain. He was a giant of a man, a stevedore with hands like spades. Culdip wanted to express sympathy. Now in England everyone knows that a hand on the shoulder is about the only non-taboo place to touch another guy. But Culdip's cultural norms led him to stroke the man's face. The shocked reaction that followed demoralised him completely. He came back to the hospice with a big bruise on his chin, asking what had he done wrong? We all fell about laughing. And the next member of the team to visit our stevedore got:

'And don't send that pouf around here no more!'

14

VOLUNTEERS – COMMUNITY SUPPORT

It is wonderful how, in towns all round the world, people have rallied to support the hospices. To receive adequate support at home there could be no one better than one's own neighbour to give it. But people are shy in offering help. Notions of not being a nuisance often make families in desperate need decline help. What we seem to need nowadays is a professional go-between who identifies the need and motivates the volunteer to serve it. Then hundreds of people come forward.

Volunteers need to be carefully screened. Interfering busybodies or people still trying to work through a bereavement themselves are excluded. A little training is needed for those who want to help with nursing care or with bereavement support.

In some well-run hospices volunteers form themselves into a team for each patient at home, working out help rotas among themselves and referring back regularly to the hospice nurse who oversees their efforts. To keep down costs many other jobs can be done in the hospice – gardening, catering, clerical work, hostessing, fund-raising, and so on. The aim is to be able to offer the hospice services free of charge at least to those families who cannot afford to contribute. We also received unpaid help from a solicitor, a pharmacist, an accountant, several doctors, clergymen and many others. Concern and help seem unlimited.

Contacting would-be volunteers involves hospice staff in lots of public lectures and meetings. Every town can and should support its own hospice, even if there is only partial support from the National Health Service. Nevertheless, the need for hospices must be constantly put before people by the

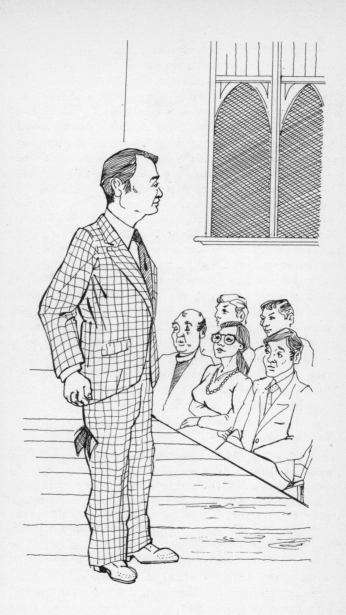

team. I was addressing such a meeting in a church hall in Newham. While answering questions I sat on the edge of the stage. A projecting nail jabbed me in the backside, so I stood up hastily, only to hear a terrifying ripping sound. A nine-inch gash in the seat of my trousers was a real tragedy because I had no money for new suits at that time, since I had not yet raised a full salary for myself. I kept talking – no one seemed to have noticed my predicament. I stiffly faced the audience for the rest of the meeting and then sidled out against the wall at the end.

Our most sterling help came from a group of cabbies who provided luxury transport to the tea parties for patients from all over the area. Volunteers also provided the refreshments and a cheery welcome in the clinic. The Christmas Week clinic was always a special event held in the Hospice conference hall. Thirty or forty patients, with their relatives, were invited. The taxis plied non-stop to get everyone to us, and then away on the dot at 4 p.m. before patients got too tired. One year the cabbies, marshalled by one of their number called Alan Fisher, decided to do even more. They staged a variety performance to entertain our guests. It was based on the Ovaltinies Show of Radio Luxembourg fame. Four cabbies in gym-slips cavorted and sang and clowned to everyone's delight.

Alan had written articles for us and was forever enlisting other people to help. Recently he wrote me a letter in which he reminisced about the years of help he gave. There was one incident in particular:

> I must tell you one little story. Three or four years ago a male patient was telling me that he would like to go on holiday with another patient and did I think that you would mind? I told him to ask you and that I was sure you wouldn't object if you thought that he was fit enough. 'Oh no' he replied, 'I know Dr Lamerton won't mind *me* going, but my friend is a woman. We'll be having separate rooms of course. Do you think Dr Lamerton will say anything?' They were both over seventy years old!

So our clinic was the seedbed of romance as well.

The counselling aspect of the volunteers' input can be a very important one. With guidance from the social worker it can develop into a major component of the hospice's contribution. In some services it has led to volunteers being included in team meetings and on boards of management.

In many cities throughout the world the Hospice League of Friends has become the principal focus of goodwill and neighbourly support. The goodness that a hospice can bring out of people and channel into urgently needed service can bring a whole community alive. In countries like South Africa, Zimbabwe and Deep South USA this has also built bridges which have contributed significantly to inter-racial harmony.

———

I sat one day in the little park at the tip of the Isle of Dogs watching the waters of the grey Thames. A glowing reflection, constantly ruffled and reforming in the swift-flowing water was cast by the stately frontage of Greenwich Palace. Domes and white colonnades tell East London of Christopher Wren its architect, and Queen Anne, his great patroness. Kings and Princes have lived in this magnificent place adorned and decorated by the nation's best artists. The Isle of Dogs is the last place where you would expect to come upon this grand view – one of the noblest and most breathtaking in Europe. And yet' 'the Island' has always been a close-knit Cockney community with a great sense of belonging, of roots. I reflected on the hospice's contribution to this atmosphere: we had cared for dozens of people in this part of Tower Hamlets.

We came at a time when tower blocks and sterile straight lines and blank concrete surfaces were replacing the maze of streets, shops and mudbanks. People whose families had lived and worked together for generations suddenly found themselves regrouped. Now it is common to find families who cannot even tell you the names of the other people living on their floor of the flats. The lifts are vandalised and stink, because people' sense of responsibility which used to embrace everyone on the street, now stops at the front door.

In fact, I had to help one old man to burgle his own flat – he was nimble enough in his seventies to squeeze through a small window – when he locked himself out. Twenty years ago a neighbour would have had a spare key. Fifty years ago it wouldn't have occurred to him to lock it.

But community is not wholly dead on the Island, thanks to the pubs and the enduring Cockney spirit. And here we were helping to revive it – bringing caring back into the home where it belongs, appealing for volunteers, asking neighbours to help, we are part of the process of this community finding its feet again after the devastating post-war social planning. It was a great privilege.

15

AN INTERNATIONAL MODEL – THE HOSPICE MOVEMENT

What we unwittingly did, in that polluted, overcrowded, lively world bounded by Dick Whittington's milestone, Spurs' football ground, Barking Creek, Tower Bridge and St Pancras's pinnacled station, was to delineate a general human need. The trail that was blazed from St Christopher's Hospice by Dame Cicely Saunders is not limited to London, Europe or even this century.

That is because it is a response, not a brain-child. The early hospices were not imposed on London: they grew, serving needs as they arose. Most human beings prefer to die in their own homes rather than in an institution. If it is not to be a harrowing experience, the family needs support. Some of this must be professional help which is essential for manipulating drugs, dressing ulcers or helping families torn apart by anger. But it would be uneconomic to have all the support given by expensive professionals, so volunteers are needed. And who better than people from the patient's own neighbourhood? In some cases patients cannot stay at home because their families cannot cope. Since hospitals – anywhere on earth – are inappropriate places for dying people, somewhere more peaceful, providing special skills and a special atmosphere is needed. That's all the hospice building really is. Suffering doesn't stop when the patient dies, and we now know that the worst complications of bereavement can be averted by good follow-up. So a bereavement service is needed. An obvious duty is to teach these skills to doctors, social workers and nurses everywhere, so hospices need teaching departments. (It is now evident that they will never do more than raise professional people's consciousness of the needs of dying patients. The fond hope of the 1980 Wilkes Report that the hospices might educate themselves into redundancy was unrealistic.)

Quite simply, this amounts to a *response* to the human condition. It isn't someone's clever programme. A service is the opposite of a programme. It is simple and logical. No more is needed and no less will do. Alas, some people who are afraid that it sets the targets too high are watering this service down, sending out unsupported nurses with no proper team to back them, or running pseudo-hospices with no home care or bereavement follow-up, or missing out vital elements like a doctor, volunteers or a social worker. Then they get together in conferences to worry why their inadequate efforts make them so depressed.

Provided all the needs of the community are met, however, the hospice model can be totally flexible. In South Africa a hospice group concluded that in Soweto one would need very little of the home care component, but in Bulawayo in Zimbabwe we heard now the support from the extended family is so good that an in-patient facility would probably never be needed. Rural settings like the American Mid-West or Lincolnshire call for utterly different approaches from big city environments like Glasgow or New York. Rich places like Zürich will use very different apparatus from poor ones like Bombay, small island communities like Bermuda will have different needs from those in seething cities like Osaka, Japan. But from all these places I have met people lit up by the hospice inspiration. And when I visit a good hospice, I know at once. The atmosphere in Te Omanga, New Zealand or Orange, Texas; the teamwork in Port of Spain, Trinidad, or Strathcarron, Scotland or San Diego, USA; the quality of volunteer commitment in Des Moines, Iowa or Melbourne, Australia, and many others, are the same. The fiery delight of service, with its distinctive hospice flavour is recognisable across the barriers of geography, language and culture. A world-wide brotherhood of friends has grown up, passionately devoted to terminal care. In Montreal, Oxford or Geneva conferences are typified by common sense and solid acvhievement, with a remarkable ease of communication and unanimity of purpose. Nothing unites people like a willingness to serve.

———

It is in this context that my little stories of East London are told. It is here at the coal-face, where real people are coping with real life problems – in all their hilarity and tragedy – that the real work is done. And there are so many stories that I haven't told. For instance, there was a patient whose headache had led to suspicions of his cancer spreading to the brain but whose actual diagnosis turned out to be after-effects from blowing up too many Royal Jubilee balloons. One man with a serious insomnia problem because I thought I was reassuring him when I said he would die peacefully in his sleep. There was the night I found myself searching for a body by torchlight in a deserted undertaker's premises and the occasion when, stuck in the lift in Ronan Point and hollaring for help, I heard two young women discussing my plight:

'Ere, do you think someone's stuck in the lift?'

'I'm not sure. I'm off Sharon, I don't want to get involved.'

'But 'e must be scared, shouldn't we tell someone?'

'Who? No Sharon, I'd leave well alone,' and off they went.

Tradition dictates that at a Jewish funeral the Rabbi, in company with the dead Jew's menfolk, solemnly heaves the first shovelful of earth into the open grave. We had one who fell in himself. Once an undertaker who was late for a funeral set off at a spanking pace in the hearse and lost the entire cortège somewhere in Hackney.

One lovely lady was called Mrs Henrietta Haunts, who said to me 'It shows how I loved him, my dear, to get 'itched to a name like that.' And Mr Ponsonby-Scrope, a boiler scaler whose secret hobby was solving mathematical problems. He told me he had learnt to live with pain – but we relieved it anyway. Sister Hilda observed that he was 'living in sin' with his girlfriend and ended the sentence with 'and he needs a urinal'.

Of course I could go on. Thirteen years in East London provided a rich experience. When I finally left St Joseph's to help launch the New Age Hospice in Houston, Texas, it was quite a wrench. The problems were the same, the needs opened one's heart in the same way, and the people were just as wonderful, but there was a certain homesickness for the mess of back streets, bad government and good humour of the East End. A return visit more recently took much longer than intended. 'Hang on, I just want to pop down here and see if they've built on London Fields yet. Let's just see Smithfield once more, and the 'Hand and Shears'. What about Clissold Park and that marvellous view on to Stoke Newington spire?' Looking up old friends again was a joy to be savoured, especially to hear again the familiar accent 'Cor, a bit taters today ain't it? [Taters = potatoes in the ,mould = cold] I've sent me skin to get some fish and chips for us. [Skin = skin and blister = sister] What was yer doin' in this 'ere Texas then?'

For me no life could have been more fulfilling, more fascinating or more fun. I meet nurses especially, but also increasing numbers of doctors, who are repelled by all the technology and paperwork involved in hospital practice, and disillusioned by the standards in so much of the National Health Service where patients' problems are often dismissed with only superficial palliatives. 'I just want to get back to good bedside nursing and spend time with patients,' they say, and come to work in a hospice.

Nursing, social work, geriatrics, disabled Olympics and many other great awakenings in the wide world of service had their origins in Britain. And now hospice care has been developed here and given to the world. I am so grateful to have been one of the spiritual children of so great a visionary as Cicely Saunders. May her work continue and with God's blessing prosper, till no one on earth need die in pain beyond the reach of a hospice team.

A SELECTION OF BRITISH HOSPICES

BATH, Avon
Dorothy House, 162 Bloomfield Road, BA2 2AT. Tel. 0225-311335 Home Care and 0225-318368 In-Patient.

BELFAST
Northern Ireland Hospice, Somerton House, 74 Somerton Road, BT 15 3LH. Tel. 0232-773735.

BIRKENHEAD, Merseyside
St John's Hospice, Mount Road, Bebington, L63 6JE. Tel. 051-334-2778.

BIRMINGHAM
St Mary's Hospice, Raddlebarn Road, Selly Park, B29 7DA. Tel. 021-472-1191.

BLACKPOOL, Lancashire
Trinity, the Hospice in the Fylde, 153/5 Devonshire Road, FY3 8BQ. Tel. 0253-301279.

BOURNEMOUTH, Dorset
Macmillan Unit, Christchurch Hospital, Fairmile Road, Christchurch, BH23 2JX. Tel. 0202-486361.

BRIGHTON, East Sussex
Coppercliff, 74 Redhill Drive, BN1 5FL. Tel. 0273-504842.

Tarner Home, Tilbury Place, BN2 2GY. Tel. 0273-604665.

BRISTOL, Avon
St Peter's Hospice, Tennis Road, Knowle, BS4 2HG Tel. 0272-774605.

CAMBRIDGE
Arthur Rank House, Brookfields Hospital, 351 Mill Road, CB1 3DF. Tel. 0223-245926.

CANTERBURY, Kent
Pilgrims' Hospice, 56 London Road, CT2 8JY. Tel. 0227-59700/57766.

CHELTENHAM, Gloucestershire
Sue Ryder Home, Leckhampton Court, Leckhampton, GL53 0AL Tel. 0243-30199.

COLCHESTER, Essex
St Helena Hospice, 22 Crouch Street, CO3 3ES. Tel. 0206-574995.

CRAWLEY, West Sussex
St Catherine's Hospice, Malthouse Road, RH10 6BH. Tel. 0293-547333.

EASTBOURNE, East Sussex
St Wilfrid's Hospice, Millgap House, 2 Millgap Road, 000 000. Tel. 0323-644500.

EDINBURGH
St Columba's Hospice, Challenger Lodge, Boswall Road, EH5 3RW. Tel. 031-551-1381.

GLASGOW
Hunters Hill Marie Curie Home, Belmont Road, G21 3AY. Tel. 041-558-2555.

GLOUCESTER

Basil Guy Foundation, c/o Mrs J. Kirkwood, Lords Meade, Longney, GL2 6SW. Tel. 0452-720349. Home Care only.

GUILDFORD, **Surrey** ALDERSHOT, **Hampshire**

Phyllis Tuckwell Memorial Hospice, Trimmers, Waverley Lane, Farnham, Surrey GU9 8BL Tel. 0252-725814.

HALIFAX/HUDDERSFIELD, **West Yorkshire**

Overgate Hospice, 30 Hullen Edge Road, Elland, HX5 0QX. Tel. 0422-79151.

HAVERING, **Essex**

St Francis' Hopsice, The Hall, Broxhill Road, Havering-atte-Bower, Romford, RM4 1QH. Tel. 0708-753319.

HEREFORD

St Michael's Hospice, Bartestree, HR1 4HA. Tel. 0432-851000.

KEIGHLEY, **West Yorkshire**

Manorlands Sue Ryder Home, Oxenhope, BD22 9HU. Tel. 0535-452308.

LEEDS, **West Yorkshire**

St Gemma's Hospice, 329 Harrogate Road, Moortown, LS17 6QD. Tel. 0-532-693231.

Wheatfields Hospice, Grove Road, Headingley, LS6 2AE. Tel. 0532-787249.

LICHFIELD, **Staffordshire**

St Giles' Hospice, Whittington WS14 9LH. Tel. 0543-432031.

LINCOLN

St Barnabas' Hospice, 17 Lindum Terrace, LN2 5RT. Tel. 0522-24145.

LONDON

St Christopher's Hospice, 51/59 Lawrie Park Road, Sydenham, SE26 6DZ. Tel. 01-778-9252.

St Joseph's Hospice, Mare Street, Hackney, E8 4SA. Tel. 01-985-0861/3.

Trinity Hospice, 30 Clapham Common North Side, Clapham, SW4 0RN. Tel. 01-622-9481.

North London Hospice, 76 Wilton Road, N10 1LT. Home Care Only. Tel. 01-444-2146.

GREATER MANCHESTER

St Ann's Hospice, St Ann's Road North, Heald Green, Cheadle, SK8 3SZ. Tel. 061-437-8136/7.

St Ann's Hospice North, Peel Lane, Little Hulton, Worsley, M28 6EL. Tel. 061-702-8181.

MIDHURST, **West Sussex**

Douglas Macmillan Unit, King Edward VII Hospital, GU29 0B2. Tel. 073081-2341

MILTON KEYNES, **Buckinghamshire**

Hospice of Our Lady and St John, The Priory, Willen, MK5 9AB. Tel. 0980-663636.

NEWPORT, **Isle of Wight**

Earl Mountbatten House, Fairlie Hospital, H29 4PT. Tel. 0983-529511/529536.

NEWPORT, **Gwent**

St David's Foundation, Cambrian House, St John's Road, Maindee, NPT 8GR. Tel. 0633-281811. Home Care and Day Care only.

NORWICH **Norfolk**
Priscilla Bacon Lodge, Colman Hospital, Unthank Road, NR2 2PJ. Tel. 0603-28377, Ext. 7241.

NOTTINGHAM
Hayward House, City Hospital, Hucknall Road, NG5 1PB. Tel. 0602-608111.

OXFORD
Sir Michael Sobell House, The Churchill Hospital, Headington, OX3 7LJ. Tel. 0865-64841, Ext. 7088.

Helen House, 37 Leopold Street, OX4 1QT. Tel. 0865-728251. Children only.

PLYMOUTH, **Devon**
St Luke's Hospice, Dean Cross Road, Plymstock, PL9 7AZ. Tel. 0752-41172.

ROCHESTER, **Kent**
Wisdom Hospice, St William's Way, ME1 2NU. Tel. 0634-812571.

ST. AUSTELL, **Cornwall**
Mount Edgcumbe Hospice, Porthpean Road, PL6 6AB. Tel. 0726-65711.

SHEFFIELD, **South Yorkshire**
St Luke's Nursing Home, Little Common Lane, Off Abbey Lane, Sheffield 11. Tel. 0742-369911.

SOUTHAMPTON, **Hampshire**
Countess Mountbatten House, Moorgreen Hospital, Botley Road, West End, S03 3JB. Tel. 0703-477414.

STIRLING/FALKIRK, **Stirlingshire**
Strathcarron Hospice, Randolph Hill, Fankerton-by-Denny, FK6 5HJ. Tel. 0324-826222.

STOKE-on-TRENT, Staffordshire
Douglas Macmillan Home, Barlaston Road, Blurton, ST3 3NZ. Tel. 0782-317118.

SWANSEA, West Glamorgan
Ty Olwen Hospice, Morriston Hospital, West Glamorgan, SA6 6NL. Tel. 0792-790112.

SWINDON, Wiltshire
Prospect Foundation, Prospect House, 5 Church Place, SN1 5EH. Tel. 0793-481458. Home Care and Day Care only.

TORQUAY Devon
Torbay and South Devon Hospice, Rowcroft House, Avenue Road, TQ2 5LS. Tel. 0803-211656.

TUNBRIDGE WELLS, Kent
Hospice at Home, Michael Tetley Hall, Sandhurst Road, TN2 3JS. Tel. 0892-44877. Home Care only.

WARWICK
Myton Hamlet Hospice, Myton Lane, Myton Road, CV3 6PX. Tel. 0926-492518.

WORCESTER/DROITWICH, Worcestershire
St Richard's Hospice at Home, 9 Castle Street, WR1 3AD. Tel. 0905-24879.

WOLVERHAMPTON, West Midlands
Compton Hall, 4 Compton Road West, WV3 9DH. Tel. 0902-758151.

WORTHING, West Sussex
St Barnabas' Home, Columbia Drive, BN13 2QF. Tel. 0903-64222.

BOOKS I WOULD RECOMMEND

Copperman, H.(1983) *Dying at Home*, Chichester, John Wiley.

DuBoulay, S. (1984) *Cicely Saunders*, Sevenoaks, Hodder & Stoughton.

Ellis, W. (1981) *The Long Road Back*, Great Wakering, Mayhew–McCrimmon.

Lamerton, R. (1980) *Care of the Dying*, Harmondsworth, Pelican Books.

Lewis, C.S. (1961) *A Grief Observed*, London, Faber & Faber.

Saunders, C. (1983) *Beyond All Pain*, London, SPCK.

Stoddard, S. (1979) *The Hospice Movement*, London, Jonathan Cape.